PRAISE FOR

Verónica's Diary

The Journey Of Innocence

"A unique marriage of memory and imagination that lights the tricky trail from childhood to young womanhood with hope!"
— Howard G. Franklin, Author, *An Irish Experience*

"*Verónica's Diary*, details the author's unique early life in Lisbon, Portugal, spanning the 1940's through the 60's, but the angst, trauma, insights and joys of growing up are timeless and universal. A wonderful story!"
— Amalie J. Hill, Author, *Ambolaja Into the Light, and Discontinuity*

"In this first person narrative, Veronica Esagui, tells her own story, in her own voice through the ages of her youth, spinning a fascinating yarn of intrigue, resilience, control, heartbreak, and fatalism. Which culminates in a course fabric of truth that is run through, unapologetically, with a fortitudinous, glowing thread of innocence and joy. A compelling read. I look forward to the next installment."
— Sharon Martini, Author, Publisher, Dotty *Beetle Books*, a division of Lady Bird Designs LLC

"A wonderful read that provides a glimpse of another culture during times past, written from a perspective that is wonderfully Veronica's. Her personal recollections whisk the reader along a unique yet personally familiar story of a child's journey into adulthood. I can't wait for the sequel."
— Danny C. Duke, Ph.D

"A richly detailed account of people and places: Lisbon, Portugal in the mid-40's and the sweeping influences of Americana; rock and roll, movie stars... and plastic tablecloths. Tales of political unrest and personal poverty anchor Verónica's march through childhood to her arranged marriage at 18. A delightful can't-put-it-down story!"
— Susan Rich, RichWriting. Marketing Business Writer & Editor

"I really enjoyed reading *Verónica's Diary* as I learned a lot about her unique and interesting life growing up in Portugal. I was amazed how much the author can remember from her entire life. I am looking forward to reading the sequel and learn more about her arranged marriage and how it all worked out."
— Susan Booth Larson, instructor at Portland Community College and Portland State University

"I was moved by the author's description of her childhood which in many ways reminded me of my own. I wanted to grab that little girl and give her a hug. I loved the book and can't wait to read the next sequel."
— Ruth Sharkey

Verónica's Diary

The Journey of Innocence

1944-1962

Veronica Esagui, DC

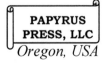

PAPYRUS PRESS, LLC
Oregon, USA

Copyright © 2010 by Veronica Esagui, DC

Library of Congress Control Number: 2010921972
ISBN 9780982648407
Second Edition
Revised and Expanded
Veronica Esagui, DC

Editors: Chory Ferguson, Maria E. Chitsaz, and John Fraraccio.

Book Cover Artist: Danlar

Illustrations: Jamie Westfall Mansilla

Graphic Designer: Derrick Villalpando

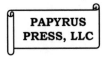

**PAPYRUS
PRESS, LLC**

21860 Willamette Drive, West Linn, OR 97068

To order additional copies of this book and or audio book

www.veronicaesagui.com

Printed in the United States of America

To my parents and Aunt Heydee,
thank you for today.

Para Lidia
con amor
Veronica Esagui DC

"*Hold on to all the experiences of growing up; someday you will need them to help you make it through life.*"

Veronica Esagui, DC

Contents

Illustrations

Lisbon as drawn by Verónica.

Preface

USA
Oregon, Tigard
Winter of 2004

My husband Dan is sitting across from me at the desk we both share. He is busy on the Internet and I am using my brand new laptop. For the last four years Dan has been doing research work concerning dioxin emissions and other toxic chemicals to which he was exposed to in Japan, while serving in the U.S. Navy. The government and the Veterans Administration are not offering any help and try to ignore his case. But Dan is very much like me; he will fight for his rights and he is not about to give up.

We have been married approximately one-and-a-half years. Dan is my best friend, and as such I always feel comfortable interrupting his train of thought to confide in him.

"I am not sure that I should change anything I wrote over the years. I realize now that the way I felt forty or even twenty years ago is not how I feel about many things today, but I probably should leave it as it is."

He responded as if thinking out loud, "I agree with that. The only difficulty I see is for anyone to believe you remember so much that happened at such a young age; most of us don't have that kind of memory."

"My goodness," I said to him, flabbergasted, as if suddenly hit by lighting, "my past life would have been a foggy time of uneventful forgotten memories, if it weren't for my mother. I can't believe it has taken me this long to realize it. While growing up I was like a sponge - when it

XV

came to catching children's diseases. It didn't matter if I got a vaccine or not. I had chicken pox, mumps, influenza, strep throat, measles, whooping cough, rubella, smallpox, a half a dozen times per year of the flu, and let's not forget tuberculosis, and having my tonsils yanked out. Yes, I was bedridden quite often and it was during those times my mother would bring me the family photo albums to my bedside. Those thick photo albums were my only source of entertainment while lying in bed recovering from whatever ailed me. Looking at each picture over and over again it became easy to recall the moment it was taken, including the previous events leading to that particular photo and what followed. The past is gone, that's true, but the diary has kept it alive. Therefore I am leaving this diary as it was intended, from the beginning as it happened, and as I perceived it then. How odd it is that I have come to this discovery of all days to pick from, today December 5? If Mama was still alive, today would be her birthday."

Author's notes

Verónica with an accent on the letter o is being kept throughout this diary as it was originally written in Portuguese.

In the diary sequel, *Braving a New World,* my full name will then change like so many other people have done, after immigrating to America.

The people and the stories portrayed in this book are all true as to my recollection when I began writing this Diary in Portuguese, Saturday, April 26, 1986 in Howell, New Jersey.

Upon translating my diary to English I have kept it as it was written, but I have changed some names to protect the not so innocent.

XVI

Spring of 1944

PORTUGAL
Lisbon
(Lisboa)

After a long and difficult night of labor, my mother finally gave birth on May 7th, a little after three in the morning. Verónica Leah Toledano Esaguy Wartenberg came out screaming her head off, as Mama described it, later on. After a week in the hospital recovering from my birth, it took a few more months at home to completely establish her health and it was during that time that my grandmother Mutter (my father's mother) took over the job of caring for me. She was the one that picked my first name; thank God for that, because my mother wanted to call me Marilia.

Summer of 1944

Grandma Mutter was born in Berlin, Germany. The stories went that she would have liked to have stayed in Portugal and continue to live with us, but the doctors in Portugal— when compared to the ones in other countries, like England — were not considered to be the best when it came to health care. Mutter was a petite, fragile-looking lady with only one kidney, but as my mother would describe her, Grandma Mutter was more like a tigress when she wanted to push her point across. Everybody agreed she was better off going to England where she had two daughters, Friedel and Ilse, along with other family members that spoke her native there was really no reason for her to stay with us.

17

Autumn of 1944

Mama did not welcome Grandma Mutter to live with us. She saw her mother-in-law taking reign of our home and family. My mother, who was born in Brazil, released her feelings towards Mutter by singing around the house a very naughty Brazilian song that vented on in-laws; *Da baia me mandaram dois presentes num bau — minha sogra jaracaca, meu sogro jarucucu.* Which means: From the bay I received two presents inside a barrel — my wacko mother-in-law and my crazy out of his head father-in-law. It sounds a lot better in Portuguese!

Mutter didn't understand much Portuguese. As a matter of a fact, she got into a lot of trouble when one day she went to the farmers market to buy some fresh fish, and asked in her best Portuguese/German accent for a big fresh *puta*. Since puta in Portuguese means a prostitute, one can imagine how those women selling fish reacted to her request.

One yelled to another, "Hey, Maria Luisa, this woman wants to buy a *puta!* Do you know anyone like that?"

Laughter became contagious, roaring like thunder down the market isles. The row of *peixeiras*, a class of working women that make a living selling fish, viciously attacked my grandmother with nasty gestures and cursing words. Mama had to rush to her rescue.

As they both walked away, one of the *peixeiras* yelled out, "If you want a big *puta* you better go downtown, that's where they hang out, my ex-husband lives with one of them."

Grandmother Mutter would not allow Mama to kiss me, unless it was my feet. She insisted that Mama's mouth carried too many germs. Mama never forgave her for that. But Grandma Mutter was not being mean; she was indeed

18

very serious about her philosophy and she wore a white starched lab coat and white gloves whenever she held me.

Tension ran high during those days of our lives and Mama cried a lot.

Winter of 1945

Grandma Mutter dressed me daily in white, soft cotton outfits and gave me daily cold baths. In the summertime it was quite refreshing I am sure, but this went on even in the winter. Mama complained to Papa that his mother was going to kill me with pneumonia, but Grandma Mutter felt this was going to be the only way that I would grow up to be a "tough cookie."

I am basically bald except for a few thin strands of black hair. I also have round fat cheeks that go along with my fat little body. I look more like a boy. But everybody praises my beauty and agrees that I look a lot like my father.

~ *Chapter One* ~

Earliest Memories

1945-1948

Spring of 1945

Walking is such an awesome, indescribable feeling. My toes are good to play with and I can chew on them when I have nothing else to do, but it's a lot more fun to stand up on my feet. In the very beginning I kept falling, but once my feet got a grip on the ground, and as long as I hold on to something, I can get to places without crawling on my knees and that is amazing!

I am one year old! I am wearing a white organdy dress with little pink and bluish butterflies sewn around the skirt and brand new white shoes — which are one size bigger than my feet, but that is good because they give me leverage to stand up. The family members and friends are gathered in our garden posing for pictures. It's my birthday today. A man with a black box on a stand keeps putting his head inside the box covered with a black cloth and his hand goes up in the air to give us the signal to stand still and smile for the camera.

A small *nespra* tree marks the center of our backyard. It was planted nine months before I was born. It needs no care, and in a few more months sweet brownish golden yellow fruits called *nespras*, will grow for our delight. The tree's green-thick leaves come in handy for grabbing onto, as I try walking around it all by myself. I am scared; no one is holding my hand and I have to rely on one of the branches closer to me within a few, but very distant, steps. Everybody is too busy talking to each other and socializing. The leaf comes off under my grasp and I fall forward on the hard sandy ground, bruising my knees. I cry. Mama calls me *chorona*, which means crybaby in Portuguese. I have not stopped crying since I left her womb, she says.

I was born with a silver spoon in my mouth, and I don't even appreciate it. I literally have it made. Papa has a very successful business, a huge delicatessen-type of German restaurant situated downtown in the chic center of Lisbon. It's a very special restaurant since it has introduced many unique items in their menu, like sauerkraut, hot dogs, butter, corn, and some traditional German dishes. The Portuguese had never experienced sauerkraut before my father opened his restaurant, and until then they had used corn only to feed the pigs.

Grandma Mutter and Grandma Rica hold each other's arms as they walk together in the garden, smiling and chatting in a mutual understanding. One doesn't speak Portuguese, the other doesn't speak German, but their French is good enough to communicate. They almost look like twins with their long black dresses and hair in the same fashion style of the day.

Mama's tummy is getting swollen and she has not been feeling good lately.

Papa held me up in his arms. Heights are very scary to me unless I am securely held tight. And I hate when someone thinks it's cute to toss me in the air and catch me midway.

Papa got busy talking to a man and his wife. I had never seen them before; he is Papa's partner in the restaurant. His wife is shy and doesn't say much. I don't like Papa's partner, and when he picked me up I grabbed his hair and tried to pull it off. He immediately put me down on the ground.

Summer of 1945

Pictures and more pictures! I do like all the attention, but I don't like the way they always prop me up in high areas from which I can fall. A good example is what happened last week, at Grandma Rica's porch. The corner of her back porch was specially set up for taking pictures. They expected me to smile, relax and open my arms without holding on to something. They seated me on top of some very shaky cardboard boxes that had been decorated with a colorful quilt over them. But I didn't feel safe, because it was high and slippery and from the corner of my eyes I could see — on my left between the iron rails — the downstairs neighbor's yard like a huge hole below me. I knew I couldn't stay up in the air, and if I fell it was going to hurt. I had fallen already several times and I know what it feels like. They wanted me to smile with the sun hitting my eyes, but that is very hard to do, because the sun makes me cry. I would rather have shade and my feet on the ground. They were very disappointed with me, I could tell.

Autumn of 1945

My brother was born today, October 9. After much dispute over which one of our grandfather's names my brother was to be honored with, they came to the mutual agreement of using both their names, Max-Leão.

Winter of 1946

I got into trouble for drinking Max-Leão's milk. I love the sweet taste of his milk bottle, but I am not allowed to drink it; Mama says I am not a baby anymore.

Spring of 1946

I am not allowed to play with Max-Leão. I was told he is a baby boy, not a doll toy. Only Mama is allowed to hold him, and that's not fair.

Summer of 1946

Our square backyard is surrounded by a whitewash-painted brick wall with a square, green, wooden door that has a wood hinge for locking; no different from the other three neighbors' backyards. Everybody in our apartment complex has a piece of land just like ours, except for the two families living on the third floor who have none. A gardener tends to the gardens, keeping the grass green and the flowers and fruit trees alive.

I like looking down from our sunroom window at the neighbor's backyard below us. They have no dirt in their yard like us. They have off-white cement walls to match the off-white cement floors. Their backyard looks like a roller-skating rink and it's always very clean. They are special.

Autumn of 1946

Blue soap for washing clothes looks like cake in a chunk, that's what attracted me to it. But I am not allowed to eat it. I don't know why. Mama yelled at me, and the maid put the soap far up in the top drawer of the kitchen closet. I can't get to it. I cry.

Spring of 1947

I looked all over the house for Grandma Mutter but she was not anywhere to be found. I looked today and yesterday in all the rooms and behind the doors and she is not here anymore. I wonder if she will be back later.

I am three years old today and Uncle Augusto came over to take pictures. What a great surprise it was! I got my own playground to play, right in our backyard! Mama and Papa had someone build me a little wooden fortress under the shade of the *nespra* tree. The fortress is a half-sawed large wooden barrel with a wood top all around it, like a tabletop.

Once inside the barrel I get to play house with the dirt, filling the tiny tin cans and tin cups with dirt and then throwing it all around me. It is a lot of fun to see the dry dirt flying all over and when I mix it with some water I can make little balls of clay and other things like dogs and cats and birds and squares. Then I mash everything together and start all over again. I love the smell of dirt and the tin cans taste very good when I lick them clean. Max-Leão is still too small to play with me.

Summer of 1947

Mama is always kissing and hugging Max-Leão. If I try to make nice to him, she will say, "Be careful, you are too rough."

You better believe that I am rough. I am also bigger than him and stronger too. I can even lift him up and it is out of kindness that I don't drop him on his head. He is kind of cute though, always smiling even when I borrow his milk bottle. I love the taste of his sweet milk formula and I hate the regular milk that I have to drink every day with my food. Besides, bottles — when turned over — don't spill the milk, and glasses do. My face hurts when I get hit across the face for being clumsy, but I can't help it, I am clumsy.

Autumn of 1947

I love playing with my little brother Max-Leão. After practicing on how to get my leverage with him on my back, I am able to carry him around the house. He doesn't mind when I drag him by the feet either. For his birthday, Mama made rice pudding. Rice pudding is not the same as cake. I refuse to eat rice with milk and sugar and a lemon peel stuck in the center of the bowl.

With a frown I say, "I want cake!"

But Mama said, "It's not your birthday! Next year, you will get a cake if that's what you really rather have."

I carefully sucked the sweet milky juice between my teeth spit the rice into my hand and little by little I stuck it under the table and under the dessert plate. It was a lot of rice to get rid of.

I saw Maria, the maid, hiding a pretty doll and a red fire truck inside one of the closets in the room next to the bathroom. I asked her about it and she said Santa Claus had asked her to hide some toys for Max-Leão and me. Next month it's Christmas. I didn't want to wait so long, and I asked Mama to tell Maria to give me the doll today. I heard the conversation in the other room. We do not believe in Santa Claus and therefore the presents are not being accepted. I cry.

Winter of 1948

Grandma Mutter's plan of making me a tough cookie failed miserably. Mama complains that I am a weakling, always sick with something or another. She is tired of constantly having to take me to her brother, Augusto. He is a doctor. She says it's almost a waste of time to treat me for anything, because as soon as I am over one sickness, I come down with another.

Chickenpox has not been easy with all the scratching, but I enjoy the warm purple baths in our big bathtub. The purple medicine in the water helps to stop the itching. Whooping cough was a lot tougher; it made me spit blood and it hurt my chest. I visit Uncle Augusto every month or so for something or another. He always smiles when he sees me because I am his favorite niece.

From the moment I was born, Uncle Augusto started taking my pictures. Every position and every facial emotion possible to a baby has been recorded by Uncle Augusto's camera. Lately things have changed a bit, since he got married and his wife had a baby, he no longer has that kind of time to spend with me, except working in the hospital or at his office. I saw his baby once, and immediately his wife blamed me for killing her child with one of my childhood diseases. But the truth is that I had nothing to do with it. Their baby died because he had something wrong with his stomach and that was the reason he vomited every time he was fed. Aunt Heydee, my mother's older sister and definitely the wisest woman I ever met, felt that his brother's wife was the one that killed the newborn, by sucking on sour candy the whole time she was pregnant and most likely giving the baby a sour stomach.

Spring of 1948

My family and I live in Lisbon, the capital city of Portugal. Our neighborhood is one of the newest and most modern areas of the city. Our building doesn't have old-fashioned tiles on the outside, it has white pinkish marble one quarter of the way up and above it is painted soft green all the way up to the third floor. Across from us on the right corner of our street there's still an empty lot of dirt where Max-Leão and I get to play once in awhile with the clay. I love playing there and I hope that no one will ever build anything on that precious ground so close to our house.

My address is Rua Ponta Delgada, # 72, first floor, on the right. Reaching the doorbell downstairs is still impossible for me. The nursemaid has to lift me up so that I can ring the bell. Max-Leão is lucky; because he is a baby he gets to ring the bell a lot more often than I. The painted green metal and glass entrance door is very wide, tall and heavy, and when it closes it makes an echoing metal noise, loud enough for everyone in the building to know it closed. This is very useful, because it lets us all know when someone has entered or left the building. Inside the hall entrance there are eight green metal mailboxes on the left wall for all eight families in our building. A very wide whitish marbled staircase, with six square marble platforms on each side, displays six lush green plants growing from six large bluish ceramic oriental pots, adorning each side of the steps. Upon reaching the top of the steps there's a small polished wood foyer, where a vase of fresh flowers sits on a small table covered with a dainty white lace cover. Usually we stop to take a break at that point and then climb three more flights, of shiny, always fresh-smelling waxed brown wooden steps covered with an Oriental rug running up the center. A matching dark-wood railing on the right side helps you to hold on. The foyer below our apartment is called the *cave* or sub-floor. The porter's apartment is below the sub-floor and their apartment doesn't have any windows. You can't go any lower than that; otherwise you reach the center of the world. That's the way most apartment houses in Lisbon are built. I feel sorry for the neighbors on the so-called second and third floor above us, they have a lot more climbing than we do.

My Grandma Rica also lives in the first floor of her apartment house and, like us, her apartment also has a sub-floor apartment under hers, with the porter and his family living below the sub-floor. But her building is a lot older than ours. Her building must be over one hundred years old, which is even older than my grandmother. They don't have potted plants, marble floors, or cork covered walls like we do; instead their wood is dull and the hallway up the steps is dark and smells like an old ship, at least that's the way I imagine it, since I have never been on an old ship, not even a new one. You can always count on lots of steps where our cousins and uncles and friends live.

Mama visits everybody, every week, and sometimes I get to go with her, so I have a lot of experience with climbing. The thick wood front door to our apartment is tall and green with a hole to see out of. There's a small bench inside that I climb on to see who is knocking. I have to look first before opening the door, in case they are robbers. Inside our vestibule we have a very tall dark-wood piano, and a small antique dresser. A medium size, black wooden owl hangs on the wall facing the front door as you come in. It belonged to

Grandma Mutter. I was almost three years old when she left for England to live with her daughters Ilse and Friedel. According to her and all the German people, owls bring you good luck, so she left it for us. Mama doesn't like the owl; she says it gives her the creeps, but just in case it's true about bringing good luck, she won't take it down. I would love to remember Grandma Mutter's face, but I don't. I feel sad that all I recall is white cotton, white lace and the smell of mothballs.

It's my birthday tomorrow. Mama is in the hospital. The maid told Max-Leão and I that it looks like we are getting another brother or sister very soon.

My new baby brother came home today. He will be the last baby Mama will have. She has sworn to that. In order to save her and the baby, Uncle Augusto and cousin Marcus, the other doctor, had to cut Mama's belly open to take our little brother José out, and then they sewed it up with a needle and thread, not much different than sewing a ripped skirt or a blouse. I am glad that I am not a doctor; it must be very difficult to sew people while they are screaming with pain.

I got a birthday cake today, a large rag doll, boxes that fit into each other, and different size blocks to make houses. Mama didn't forget my birthday, she was just too sick from having José taken out of her tummy and then having to carry him home from the hospital last month. I like my toys, but I wish I had a pretty doll like the one Maria was going to give me for Christmas instead of this big limp one made of cloth. But I am happy that my cousins came over and they had rice pudding but I didn't have to eat it. Mama remembered her promise from last year and I had my own little personal birthday cake with four candles.

Summer of 1948

Max-Leão and I share our bedroom. It doesn't have a window to the outside like the other rooms, but we have a narrow, horizontal window close to the ceiling that opens from our bedroom to the Imperial Room, as Mama calls it, because it is decorated with golden furniture. We like the little window above us because in the summer it provides some form of fresh air even if it doesn't come from the street, and we also get to listen to adults talk in the other room, which helps us to fall asleep quicker.

We have two doors to our bedroom; one is our normal regular door to enter the room from the vestibule, the other a French- style door that opens to our parent's bedroom right next to ours. When Mama or Papa comes to hit us, we use these doorways to run away from them. Around and around I run, from one room to the other, for as long as I can, from our bedroom through their bedroom and out into the vestibule. I have gotten pretty good around the curves, a few extra painless minutes of my life, and even though I can run very fast, sooner or later I get caught when Mama or Papa extend their long arms and grab me.

Their bedroom furniture is very pretty; the two armoires are opulent, tall, and wide, made of golden wood with mother-of-pearl inlaid flowers around the mirrored doors and the side panels, matching the vanity fair of three mirrors. Most of our furniture came from Germany. José sleeps in our parent's bedroom because he is always sick. The other bedroom facing the street is the guest room and Grandma Rica or one of Mama's sisters gets to use it when they stay with us overnight. When Grandma Rica is sick, she always stays with us until she is well.

In the hallway wall between the Imperial Room and the pantry there is a very large framed award written in gold around a silver medal with a centrally located seal of different colors. I like staring at it. The King of Spain gave this award to Mama, when she wrote a musical composition just for him. This happened before she met Papa. After she got married, she gave up her career to become a devoted wife and mother. Mama is very proud of how beautiful she used to be, before she met Papa and gave up her musical career for us. I like to picture her in my mind as she played the piano in the king's palace with her long dark hair parted perfectly to the side of her face and down to her shoulders, and she smiled with an air of pride as the handsome King of Spain kissed her hand and gave her the well-deserved silver medal.

The Imperial Room is a long and wide subdivided room that has a living room and dining room with lots of golden furnishings. It's used for special occasions only, like company or parties. Because Max-Leão and I are very clumsy and might break something, we are not allowed in that room; therefore we call it "the forbidden room."

I can remember only one time that I was allowed to have dinner with my parents and their guests, and it must have been a very special day because not only did we have the regular maids bring the food from the kitchen but we also had a man dressed in a black suit with a long-tail jacket serving us at the table. It was a very elegant experience and I had a chance to eat with silver utensils on a silver trinket. I have dreams at night about all the possibilities that could happen there if Max-Leão and I were allowed to play in that room.

A little down the hallway, on the right side, there's a built-in wall closet where Mama keeps most of our quality linen, and her antique silverware collection under lock and key. The door to this closet has four tiny holes so that air can get inside. When Mama opens it, I like to stand next to her. It is a very mysterious closet, always under lock and key.

She always says, "What are you looking at? It's nothing but linens, towels and bed sheets."

But I know that there has to be something else inside this closet, something like a hidden treasure, way in the back. There might even be another locked door, another entrance to some strange and scary place.

A few steps down on the left side of this hallway, there is a small dingy dark room without a window. This is where the full-time maid sleeps and the groceries are stored. We are not allowed in there either, which is good because it smells of spoiled rotten groceries, sauerkraut and other unidentified smells. A few more steps down the hallway is our dining room on the left side. What I find amazing in this room is the crusted thick panels on the front and sides of the old furniture reminding me of camouflaged castle doors. The table where we eat matches the furniture with its own labyrinth of holes and spaces where I can hide any food that I don't like. Bread can be squeezed right into its niches and cracks. I really don't like bread, unless it's used as a tool to push the food onto the spoon or fork, as it keeps my fingers clean. For some reason, which I have not figured out yet, there is a real glass window from our dining room to the Imperial Room. Why would anyone put a window that doesn't open to the street but instead opens from one room to another? It was probably built so that Max-Leão and I can look into the "forbidden room" without having to actually go inside.

We don't have to go far from our dining room to wash our hands, since the bathroom is right next to it. The bathroom window is always open, for fresh air, but I always close the wooden shutters when I have to use the bathroom. I don't want any of the neighbors to see my bottom before I sit on the toilet. If I forget to open the shutters again, I get yelled at. I have very poor memory. The bathroom window faces the neighbor's building next to us and from my bathroom window I can see their gardens and I can also glimpse at what they are doing if they forget to close their shutters.

Inside the bathroom there's a deep white bathtub with metal animal paws, a white bidet, a white washing basin, and a white toilet with a small straw basket right next to it, containing lots of small, neatly folded and cut pieces of newspaper for wiping yourself afterwards. Aunt Heydee says that we are lucky to have newspapers to wipe ourselves. In

Brazil, she had to use twigs or leaves from the trees, since going to the bathroom meant going outside into the woods. I wonder if ants got inside of her when she wiped herself with the tree leaves. It is a horrible thought, but a very possible one. If I were a little ant I would not know the difference between one hole and another.

When I pull on the cord with a wooden handle coming down from the tank above our heads the toilet gets flushed with water. The floor of white and black tiles is always cold and in the summer they feel good on the feet. A long Persian carpet extends through the hallway from each bedroom, and that feels wonderful in the winter. The only heat I get on cold nights is when a hot water bottle awaits between the blankets. Sometimes it's so cold in the winter that when I lay down, my teeth chatter for a long time and I try to hold off as long as possible from making wee in the middle of the night. Even though I have a handy ceramic pan under the bed it is too cold to sit on it. After using it, I slip the ceramic pan right back under the bed frame as fast as I can so that I can snuggle back into the straw mattress where my body's indentation still holds its warm shape. The next morning the maid disposes the pot's contents before she even makes the beds. Next to the bathroom is the kitchen with a smoked-glass door. If it is closed, do not enter, the cook is probably running around in circles with a knife in her hand after a headless chicken and there will be blood all over the place. Max-Leão was with me the first time we saw that happen. He fainted.

Our kitchen is very huge and has a large, light gray marble platform with a dark metal stove with lots of little doors in the front. In a corner there's a wooden closet where the maid puts chunky ice blocks in its drawers. She buys the ice from the iceman in the street. Sometimes I go with her to see the ice carriage and the horse that pulls it. The iceman is always cranky and swears a lot. Not an easy job considering that he uses a long metal stick with a hook on the tip to pull the ice off the carriage and then he breaks the ice into smaller pieces with an ax. Afterwards he has to carry the ice chunk on his shoulder to the first floor where we live.

I can always tell when the maid is cleaning the ice-box as I hear her complaining, "Taking out the melted water every so many days is a real mess, if you were to ask me, just to keep the food cold."

The kitchen has a small window that opens to the neighbors in the building next to us. This window is on the right side of the cold marble pinkish-gray sink with a wooden storage place underneath it. The sun is always shining on the kitchen sink, even on cloudy days. From the kitchen there are two sets of doors that open to the sunroom; a very large laundry, sewing, and ironing kind of room. The inner doors are made of hard thick painted white wood, with a long wooden arm that is used to secure the doors at night from inside like the front door. Those doors stay open during the day but the tall white French doors can be opened or closed depending on the need to keep cool in the summer or warm in the winter.

In this room there is an old linen closet, a big gray stone basin with ridges to wash the laundry and in the corner of the room there's a pit hole where the grease and undesirable leftovers are dumped. A round wood piece covers the pit hole and on top of it sits a round tin box that previously contained sugar cookies. It is now used for keeping the sewing needles, buttons and thread of various colors. The smell that comes from the pit is really gross. Sometimes Max-Leão and I lift the lid up to confirm that the smell coming from the pit is really the worst smell we have ever experienced. Next to it is the maid's bathroom, with a small sink and barely any space to sit on the toilet. It is literally covered with mops and tools for cleaning the house; I always wonder how they can even find enough space to use the toilet, and besides, how do they take a bath? I wonder because there's no tub. I have peeked in there a few times to see if there is space for me to hide from Max-Leão when we play hide and seek, but I have never used it, because there is no space to hide. No one has to tell us to stay away from the maid's bathroom.

Of all the rooms in our house my favorite is the sunroom. I like to sit by the large glass window that opens wide like a huge smile from wall to wall to a whole outside of neighbors and their gardens. The sky is very big from this window, and straight ahead in the distance I can see a white church on top of the hill where they play the tower bells on the hour, and on Sunday mornings and festive occasions they play church tunes. The dark brown, long building next to it is a military arsenal where they keep lots and lots of gunpowder and guns. If Spain decides to attack Portugal again, like they have done so many times in the past, we are ready to fight back.

From the sunroom there's a small green metal door that opens to a small atrium outside, and is shared with our next-door neighbor. Each of us has an outside wall closet with a green wooden door that is used for storage of goods that are delivered early in the morning by the grocery boy, the milkman, and the bread man. Nobody bothers to lock it anymore. Somehow the key got lost about a year ago. The black shiny metal stairs go all the way up to the third floor and down to the backyard below us, where it stops at the marble patio below. Two long marble staircases reach the neighbors below us and the porter's place below them. Passing by the porter's door on my left, there is a long dark stone tunnel that puts me at the back door gate and into the busy street outside. A key is needed to get back in because the door closes automatically behind us. Even though this back exit is to be used only by the maids, delivery people, and the porters, the gypsies always find their way in to ask for bread and money.

My brothers and I always have a nursemaid during the day. Usually, she is a young girl that plays with us and takes us out for walks to the park up the street and feeds us so that we are ready to get into bed by the time Papa is home from work. Mama spends most of her time visiting the family, shopping, or going out with Papa. The full-time maid takes care of the rooms, dusting and cleaning windows and waxing floors, and she runs errands and assists the cook in the kitchen. Her name is Maria and she lives with us, she sleeps in the smelly room with the groceries.

Mama took Max-Leão and I to the hospital for a blood test. The hospital smell makes me sick; I shake a lot when I go to the hospital, that's where people go when they want to feel pain and die. They took blood from my arm with a syringe and I cried a lot. Max-Leão is so smart though, he fainted and they asked Mama to come back another day with him. On the way home we took the trolley car but Max-Leão started to vomit. It was something about him being trolley car sick and we had to walk the rest of the way home. Mama carried him in her arms and I had to help by carrying her heavy pocketbook up the hill from Plaza do Chile.

I love Uncle Augusto's waiting room. In the center of the waiting room there is a large, huge dark wood table with thick curly legs that twist into a game room beneath it. It is incredible that nobody else is aware of this except Max-Leão and I. It is a puzzle to me to observe other children in the waiting room seated next to their parents or family members, and obviously not aware of this playground. Even the chairs have legs that match the table. It is an absolutely amazing maze, crawling from one chair to another under the patient's legs!

I did go willingly the first time into Uncle Augusto's treatment room, behind closed doors, because I thought he was going to take my picture, but I immediately noticed a container with various needles boiling in water over a small gas burner. After he looked into my throat and gagged me with some wooden stick, he actually expected me to drop my pants down so that he could stick me with one of his boiled needles. It seems to me that it has become a habit for my uncle to treat me for any ailment I might have with a shot every time we visit him. Mama, the nurse, and him don't seem to understand why I scream and hold on to the corners of the waiting room walls or the legs of the chairs with all my mighty strength. The only way I go into his office is by being dragged by my hair. Of course I am going to scream. All they are going to do is inject me with penicillin, and that hurts.

Max-Leão and I eat a lot of carrots while seated in the sunroom's window. Mama told us, if we eat a lot of carrots, even though neither one of us likes them, we will get pink eyes like the rabbits. It's a worthwhile sacrifice; I love pink. The sunroom is our favorite room for having fun. I like playing with buttons of different colors and feeling the different textures. Raw rice is very nice too, for making roads on the sunroom's floor. Max-Leão likes to play with his miniature cars and I like to build the roads for him. Together we make roads and hills and even dead ends. We have lots of fun playing together.

Mama took me to Papa's restaurant for the first time. It's in downtown Lisbon, on the Rua do Carmo. Women love to shop in this part of the city where everything is very beautiful and expensive. Papa greeted us at the entrance of the restaurant. He was very happy to see us. It was a surprise. He seated us at a small table overlooking the crowd seated below us having lunch. Our waiter brought us a deep crystal plate each filled with fresh strawberries covered with whipped cream. I felt very grown up but I was also nervous. I was afraid that if I dropped a strawberry on the white-linen tablecloth Mama would never take me out again. I was praised for having good table manners.

Autumn of 1948

I am starting kindergarten! Mama wants to make sure that I know my name in full, and also both my parents' names. It's so much easier to say, Mama or Papa. It's hard to remember their names. Mama told me that she is disappointed with my poor memory, I can hum a song but I can never remember the words. She made me stand up in front of her while she held José and Max-Leão, her two favorite children next to her, kissing and hugging them, and she made me repeat my name and my parent's names, our telephone number, and our address over and over again. For dinner she prepared calf brains stewed in wine, just for me. It's supposed to help with memory problems like mine. I am scared about tomorrow.

A small school van picked me up early in the morning by our front door. I am going to a private school for rich kids. As the van went from house to house, I got a chance to see the homes of other little boys and girls, along the Avenue Almirante Gago Coutinho. A long name for a street but most likely it was chosen because a short name for this road would not make any sense, as it is a long road to reach the airport. These homes are not apartment houses like ours; they are big houses, small palaces to be described more properly, in the most expensive and newest side of town. These are the children of important people in the community that are able to afford the high monthly tuition.

I love school. There are lots of toys to play with. Inside a box in the hallway there was a little game that I wanted to keep, so I took it home with me. *Why leave it there overnight, nobody can enjoy it that way*, I thought to myself as I put it in my pocket and proudly displayed it to Mama when she asked me what I had learned that day. She told me that I stole the toy!

"It's called stealing, when you take something that doesn't belong to you," she said.

I started to cry. I'm not a robber. I cried a lot but it didn't do me any good. I have to put the toy back where I took it from, tomorrow morning. Mama says that I might be going to jail if they find out what I did. What a horrible thing to happen. I just started school and I am already in trouble. If I get caught I'll be going to jail forever, never to see my family again, and worst of all I'll be forced to eat the only thing I hate, bread. I'll starve to death most likely, and without a spoon I will never be able to dig myself out of jail. I was so scared they would catch me putting the toy back in the toy box. What would I say? I robbed the school yesterday, and admit to being a criminal? After lunch when they turned the lights off so that we could all take a nap, I got up as if I was going to the bathroom. Holding tight to the labyrinth toy in the coat pocket of my gray uniform, I opened the big toy box in the hallway and then feeling like I was going to faint, like Max-Leão does so often, I dropped the toy into the box and closed it quickly. I did it! Nobody saw me.

I am learning the numbers and letters of the alphabet and I am having lots of fun making paper toys, drawing, and even sewing with wool thread little animals onto cardboard pieces. Yesterday, I didn't go to school because the whole class was sick, something to do with a boy that brought candy to school. Mama said I was the only one that didn't get sick. She said that the boy was giving out poison candy, and because I was a good obedient girl, nothing happened to me.

I didn't say anything to Mama but I think that the little boy is very nice, because he shared his candy with the ones that asked for some. The only reason that I didn't eat any candy was because he had run out of it by the time I got close enough to him. I didn't tell that to Mama. I want her to think that I was being good, like she wants me to be.

Uncle Augusto has prohibited Mama from taking me to see him during office hours because of the traumatic experience that I put his patients through. It seems that witnessing my distress and hearing my screams coming from inside his treatment room is scaring the living soul out of his patients waiting patiently in the waiting room. I am just trying to warn them of what is really going on behind closed doors. At Mama's request he gave her the needles and the penicillin so that she can give us the shots at home whenever my brothers or I get sick. I have so many lumps on my bottom now. She says it's because I move. I have to stay still so she doesn't break the needle inside my butt cheek. This should be illegal in my opinion, just because her brother is a doctor it doesn't make her a medical person. Every time we get a cold or a sore throat, we get a shot. Max-Leão has a lot more lumps on his bottom than I do. He moves more than me. Lately he's been getting daily hot compresses to make the lumps soft and melt away. We both get these lumps after Mama gives us the penicillin shots. They are the cure for everything, a miracle drug, so they say.

I found out that I have pretty eyes. I was running up the school steps when two women were coming down the steps, one pointed at me, "Look at that little girl, have you ever seen such beautiful green eyes?" I stopped for a moment and stared back at them. My face felt very hot as I ran into the school with an embarrassed but happy feeling. I am not going to eat so many carrots; green eyes make people say nice things to me.

I want to be a teacher when I grow up. When the teacher leaves the classroom, I like to climb on her chair and then to the top of her desk. From there I hold up the wooden stick and I point to the various letters of the alphabet that hang on the walls around us. Being in kindergarten is a lot of fun. A new teacher came into the classroom this afternoon; I had no idea what she was talking about until she asked us if we knew the name of the father. Well, it was about time, I thought to myself. I know the name of my father really good, but no one had asked me that yet. I raised my right hand eagerly.

"You, what's your name?" she pointed to me.

"My name is Verónica Leah Toledano Esaguy Wartenberg." I smiled to her.

"Very well, Verónica, tell the class the name of the father."

Taking a deep breath I said, "His name is Hans!" *Oops, silly me, I should say the whole name as I had learned it.* "His name is Hans Joachim Wartenberg." And I smiled again.

"Verónica, are you making a mockery of our father?"

"No," I said, surprised by her anger. "His name is Hans Joachim Wartenberg!"

"Come up here, right now, next to me." When I got near her, she pulled hard on my left ear and yelled, "The name of our Father is Jesus, now repeat it to the class!"

"No, it's not Jesus," I replied, very sure of myself, "You are wrong, his name is Hans and he is not your father."

She was very mad and would not admit that she was wrong. She hit my hands with a wooden ruler until the palm of my hands and wrists were red and then made me stand the rest of the day facing the wall. I was not allowed to go to the bathroom and I hate getting wet, what a mess!

When I got home I showed my bruised hands to Mama and told her about the mean teacher. I don't like school anymore and I don't want to go back.

That night I heard Mama talking to Papa, something about religion and God and it's about time that she took me to the temple. Papa didn't agree because he doesn't like religion; he feels it's too early to put man-made, silly-religious stuff into my head.

I may have all the illnesses of childhood, but José my little baby brother has the kind of sickness that can kill him. He gets taken to the emergency room even in the middle of the night. A few times he almost died from lack of air. Someone told Mama that high altitude is good for José, so they took him today on an airplane ride. I wish I had asthma too; it's not fair that he gets to fly and I don't.

Papa rarely talks to us. Kids are not to be seen or heard. When he gets home after work, Mama tells him how bad we behaved and asks him to hit us. At first he screams at me and that is scary enough, I already know what follows afterwards.

I try to protect myself with my hands in front of my face, but it doesn't really help, his hands are big and heavy. When he hits me across the face it stings and I feel dizzy when everything shakes inside my head. He speaks Portuguese with a very harsh accent. I can always tell when he is angry because the words are like crushing thunder sounds, except they are made with the German language. I am afraid of Papa.

I am so happy that our meals are served earlier, before Papa comes home. When we eat together on rare occasions I have to be careful not to spill my glass of milk, if I do I get slapped across the face for being clumsy.

In the evening Mama will say, "Go to Papa to get your blessing and then go to bed, it's late."

If Mama didn't ask him to punish us all the time, maybe, he would not bother with us when he gets home. He must think that my brothers and I are terrible kids and he probably hates us too.

Our nursemaid Paula was fired a few days ago. We were alone with her at home and she had Max-Leão and me sitting on the foyer floor in a ring-like format. It was kind of dark and the lights were not on. Paula was not wearing underwear and she put one of Max-Leão's fingers in her vagina and asked him to wiggle it around, but he pulled his hand out and refused to do it and cried when she yelled at him. She then asked me to put my finger in there and move it around. I didn't really want to do it but I am always being hit for not being obedient, so I did it. It felt wet and gummy, and I thought she was probably itching or something, because she wanted me to do it harder. I didn't know that was bad until Max-Leão told Mama that he didn't want to put his fingers inside Paula's vagina. He complained to Mama, because he was not happy being yelled at earlier that day. Mama fired Paula, and I was told what I had done was disgusting.

"Why is it disgusting?" I asked, "I was doing what she told me to do."

But Mama called me a bad girl and stupid too if I didn't know why it was disgusting. It seems that I'm damned if I do

42

what adults tell me to do, and I'm damned if I don't. I should hide away and not look at anyone or talk or play with anyone. I get blamed for everything, all the time.

There was a lot of odd noise coming from the Imperial Room this evening. I heard someone crying. I took a peek between the French doors. I saw Papa sitting on his armchair with his hands covering his face, and he was crying and saying over and over again, "What am I going to do now? How am I going to feed my family? What am I going to do, we are ruined!" Mama was by his side crying too.

"Don't worry, I can lend you some money, it's not much but it can help," said Aunt Heydee, Mama's sister.

Wow! Papa and Mama crying! They were crying with tears coming out of their eyes just like me. They must be in pain, just like when I get spanked. No one stopped my brothers and me from entering the Imperial Room, so we went directly to the golden Viennese armoire with glass doors displaying vases and glasses made of crystals and a golden glass with a beautiful lady's face imprinted on it. We just stayed there staring at the treasures of wondrous beauty. Then the maid came in, picked José up and ordered us to follow her into our bedrooms. I wondered what happened. Nobody would tell us why everybody was sad.

Winter of 1949

The maids are gone. I no longer can go to kindergarten school. I miss the smell of crayons and paper. I miss working with arts and crafts at school, using colorful papers and cutting them into fun pieces with plastic scissors and sewing little cards with wool thread. I miss singing French songs like *Frére Jacques*, and English songs like *London Bridge Is Falling Down*, while dancing along with the other children. It looks like we are on our own from now on.

~ Chapter Two ~

Dandelions in the Garden

1949-1950

Spring of 1949

When I walked in the kitchen this morning, Mama was pulling her hair and screaming as she cried out, "Now they are taking our bathtub!" Two men were carrying it out the kitchen's back door. Each day something is being sold to make ends meet. She was hugging my brothers as she cried; I stood against the kitchen door looking at her. I didn't understand the magnitude of what was happening. I walked slowly towards her, not quite sure of what to do to console her. She called me to come closer to her and she hugged me too. We all held on to Mama, hoping she would stop crying. The next-door neighbor came by and said she was sorry about what she had heard. Papa lost his restaurant on account of his partner stealing from him. It had to do with his partner making bad checks, and other matters that I don't understand. The fact was that Papa is in a lot of trouble. His partner ran off with his family to another country, the United States of America, and he left no address. He is nowhere to be found. He had everything well planned in advance. I hope he dies when he gets to America.

There are no furnishings left in our house; most everything has been sold. Except for my parent's bedroom furniture and our beds, the house is empty. The stove is gone too. The Imperial Room is now one long empty room, and we can play in it. The months ahead are going to be difficult, mostly borrowing money from family members since no one will hire Papa to work. The Jewish community is no help; he is a German, and therefore a Nazi. The Portuguese will not hire him, because he is a Jew. He killed Jesus Christ.

Whenever I am bedridden, Mama brings me a couple of the family albums so I don't get bored. Sometimes she tells me the stories connected with the older pictures, the family members that I never met and how they came about. Looking at these pictures a couple of times per year, depending on how soon I get sick, keeps me busy until I get better. With each picture I can hear and feel its moment drawn out of the photo album as it felt before and after each picture was taken. No words are needed. The pictures are loud and clear, twirling in the windmills of the past, connecting with the present and still looking forward to the future, like a magic carpet promising to return each time, for as long as I am sick.

Old bread is not so bad when it boils in water with garlic for a while, and by adding fresh parsley, which is free when you buy the garlic, the soup can taste like real food. Sometimes an egg is available, and dinner becomes a real treat. I also developed a taste for bread with *yummy* raw onions. Besides, I want to grow very old like my Grandma Rica so that I can have wrinkled hands like hers. Mama told me that Grandma eats a lot of onions and that's why she is still alive.

For my birthday Mama bought me a cupcake; she knows I don't like rice pudding. She said it is very important to have a cake and candles to blow on your birthday. Right now, a cupcake is a luxury.

I don't like getting constantly beat up for things when I don't even understand the reason why. A few weeks ago I tried to show Mama what it feels like getting hit. I followed her down the hallway and then very quickly I tapped on her backside. I wanted her to understand how it feels, and she should stop hitting me all the time. I did it very delicately, but she is too smart for me, she realized right away my intentions and she turned around and said, "You dare to hit your own mother? This is what you get!" And she hit me so hard that I went flying into the wall resulting in a bloody nose. The whole idea of teaching her, a lesson failed miserably. I am not even going to try it on Papa.

I asked Mama, "Why don't I have a penis like my two brothers? What's wrong with me?"

She put a carrot on a string and tied it around my waist, saying, "Ok, now you have one too."

What's the matter with Mama, can't she see that I don't want a carrot or a penis; I just want to know why I am different?

There was a crystal, bluish-tinted bottle of perfume in the top shelf of the closet in the room next to the bathroom. Max-Leão and I had our eyes on it for quite a while. We wanted to see it more up close. I got up on a chair and brought it down. We both took a sniff and agreed that it smelled really good! But my brother decided that something that smelled that good had to be very tasty too. He started to drink it and I tried to take it away from him but he would not share it with me. He drank the whole bottle of perfume and Mama got home just in time to rush him to the hospital where they pumped his stomach. I am the oldest and therefore I am supposed to know from life's experience that I had given poison to my brother to drink. The punishment is always the same, a lot of screaming, getting hit across the face or having to pull my underwear down so that I can feel more pain when Mama puts me over her knees and hits my bottom with a wood spoon. As if that was not enough punishment she always adds, "Wait until your father gets home."

Max-Leão and I got into trouble today. We got caught using cockroaches for racing down the hallway. It's easy to find big ones. They are everywhere. We have been doing that since our hallway carpet was sold. We use the hardwood floor strips for racing them. We put the cockroaches side by side at the beginning of the hallway and then we wait to see which one gets to the end of the hallway first. Since we are not allowed to play with the roaches anymore, we have to wait until Mama is out with José. Mama put cucumber skins on the ground outside the front door to our apartment and also by the back door, so the roaches can't come in from either direction. Someone told her roaches don't like cucumbers. But it doesn't look like they are using the front or back doors to come in. They must be coming in through the little holes in the walls. Mama says they are coming in from the neighbor's next door, where else could they be coming from? We keep our apartment clean and they still come into our apartment. We don't have a way of stopping them, there's too many of them. I would love to have mice instead, like at Grandma Rica's old house. They are so adorable. Everybody screams when they see them running in and out of little tiny holes on the walls, but I find them to be very cute fuzzy little creatures.

All our toys are gone; Mama put everything into a sack and said she was giving them away to needy children. I have a feeling that she is selling them, like everything else we have.

I don't play with roaches anymore. I can't even think of it without getting the willies. Now that Mama said my brothers and me are too old to have a pot under the bed, we have to get up during the night to use the bathroom. I have started turning the hallway lights on this week, so the roaches will run away and I won't step on one of them with my shoes. The crunching sound is just too much for me.

It all started when I got up one night barefoot in the dark and somewhere halfway down the hall I stepped on a huge roach. Thick white blood and guts came out of it. I had to wash my right foot in the bidet, because we have no tub and the washing basin is too high for me to get my foot inside.

I love going to Grandma Rica's house. We are there very often for dinner. We also go there to bathe in her chipped enamel tub, which is very large and much deeper than the one we used to have; it looks like a metal boat. Grandma Rica was born in Tangier, Morocco where she learned to make special jams with grapes and other fruits like apples. She also makes orange skin covered with chocolate. Everything is stored in her cool-dark pantry room with other unusual delicacies. When Grandma Rica gives me a banana and bread I eat the banana and throw away the bread. I only eat bread if there's nothing else to eat. My favorite meal is fava beans with meatballs or sweet peas with meatballs. When Aunt Heydee makes the food, there aren't much fava beans left, only meatballs. She keeps testing the fava beans as they cook. "Just making sure they don't get overdone," she says.

Aunt Heydee lives with her mother Rica, and so does Aunt Ligia, her youngest sister. I like to sit next to them and listen to their stories. Ligia is a very nervous and neurotic person. She was in a mental institution for a while. She had to have electric shock treatments to make her forget some emotional trauma she suffered a few years ago. I am going to try my very best never to go crazy like her, since the idea of electric shocks is very scary. She was to be married when, one week before the wedding, her fiancée changed his mind and Aunt Ligia had a nervous breakdown. She even tried to kill herself. A few years later she got married to someone else but he used to beat her up and she got a divorce. Everybody feels her ex-husband was a bad man because he was not a Jew. Jews love their wives and never beat them. The whole thing was her fault. Now she is divorced and alone with two children from that marriage and living with Grandma, until she can afford to be on her own. She is a poetess and writes children stories and also writes for the main newspaper in Lisbon, the *Diário de Notícias*. She started writing when she was fourteen years old; *The Sin* was never published but in 1942 her first book *Him* was published and the year after *Her*

was published. She loves to write. At present she is writing two other books, *Those Kisses*, a poetry book, and the novel, *Bodies for Sale*. When she is not writing, which is rare, she teaches gymnastics at a high school, trying to make ends meet.

Papa found a job. He is now selling magazines and books from door to door. He climbs a lot of steps up and down apartment complexes in the city of Lisbon, and he carries in each hand one large suitcase filled with books and magazines about architecture and art. Some days he sells a few of them; sometimes he comes back with what he started with. When he gets home he is always very tired and his chest hurts. Breathing becomes difficult when his chest hurts. Cousin Salomão, who is a cardiologist, diagnosed Papa with a heart disease that kills you when you exert yourself. Papa can die anytime, and should not be straining himself climbing steps and carrying heavy books but he is the only breadwinner in our family.

The German gold wine glass with the painted face of a lady is back on the shelf in one of the armoires. It never got sold. Mama picked it up from the pawnshop where she gets money for leaving it there until she has enough money to get it back.

Summer of 1949

Mama has been cooking. She creates food with what is available, which can be a horrible experience. But her cookies are very good, even if they are hard as a rock. They just have to be soaked in hot milk or we will break our teeth. They always smell so incredibly delicious, the vanilla and orange make my mouth water every time. Last week, Max-Leão and I were throwing them at each other and one of them scratched José's head ever so slightly but kept on going and broke the glass window in the kitchen closet. Both Max-Leão and I can't sit down at all.

Mama woke me up early in the morning to go to the Santa Cruz hospital with her. Supposedly she had to see her doctor. Usually we go to Uncle Augusto's office where she takes diathermy treatments for her tummy, because once a month her tummy hurts a lot. She would not tell me much about this visit to the hospital. She is always very mysterious about everything. While walking to the hospital I hopped up and down like I do when I feel happy and I ran up in front of her humming a few tunes. When crossing the street I held her hand. I was happy to go out with Mama.

We entered the stagnant, smelly, hot hospital's large waiting room packed tight with sick people. There were no fun tables or chairs to run under, like in Uncle Augusto's office. There were a lot of children in the waiting room, some were sneezing, others were coughing, and that weird acid-like smell I hate, the hospital's smell of blood and tincture of iodine and chemicals were all around us. I have noticed that the mortuaries, with saints made of wax and candles of all sizes, are always close to the hospitals.

We didn't wait long; a woman dressed in a long white coat with grayish hair pulled back tight, thick glasses, and a frowned face, asked me to go with her.

I looked at Mama questioningly and she just said, "Go with the nurse. I'll be waiting here for you."

I followed the nurse as I was told, but as soon as I entered the room behind closed doors I knew I was in trouble. I ran for the door but the gray-haired woman grabbed me from the back of my dress. I started to scream and called out for Mama to help me. Two other men in white coats came to help her. I kicked them in the shins as hard as I could and they got very angry and dragged me to a chair, while someone else tied my legs down. With my arms held behind my back by the nasty woman and some other nasty mean people, they asked me to open my mouth to a man with some kind of round light bulb on his forehead and a pair of pliers in his hand who also impatiently asked me to open my mouth. No way was I going to open my mouth! But then they squeezed my nose and held my head still between their hands and arms and they pulled my hair back. I had to open my mouth in order to breathe. As they held my jaw open, one of the men in white coats started cutting the inside of my throat off with pliers. It was hard to breathe and blood was coming out and I was gagging from it. Then they let me free. I came out of the room and Mama just took me out by the hand outside to the street. I wanted to ask Mama why this happened to me but I couldn't talk and she was not talking to me either. She didn't even ask me what happened. Obviously she had taken me there on purpose. What could I have done wrong to deserve such punishment?

She waited for a taxi to go by, and we got in, while I held to my mouth the handkerchief she gave me, blood was coming out of my mouth. When we got home she put me in bed. She didn't hug or kiss me. I was crying, in pain and with no idea of what had just happened. Then she said, "You just had your tonsils out, now you won't be so sick anymore." And she added, "God punished you, for being happy that your mother was going to the hospital."

I wanted to talk and defend myself from such accusations that I felt were completely untrue, but I couldn't make a sound. I wanted to tell her that I hated her for lying to me. And then she offered me vanilla ice cream. I felt she was doing that on purpose, since I could not even swallow my own spit and I hated her. The only thing that I am happy about is that my bedroom is now in the front room of the house, where the sun comes in and lights it up. Mama told me that tomorrow I can try and eat ice cream since my throat will not hurt anymore.

Autumn of 1949

We have been eating our meals in the kitchen since we don't have a dining room set anymore. Mama got a table and some chairs from Grandma Rica and someone gave us loose pieces of plywood to put over the cold tile floor in the kitchen. This way, when it gets colder in the winter, our feet won't freeze and give us a bladder virus. Mama says that's what happens if your feet get too cold. The room where we used to have our meals before we became poor is now a playroom. My two brothers and I play in there, but there are no toys to play with. The room is empty. Before locking us in the room, Mama tells us to use our imagination. We jump up and down to see who can jump the highest, and when we get tired we sit on the floor and tell each other scary stories. My brother José doesn't do much of anything but drink milk from his bottle. He is about a year and a half old and is still in diapers. He is too small for anything much but watching us. When we run out of imagination, Max-Leão and I try to bite each other's bottom by grabbing each other around the waist and going around in circles.

The neighbor downstairs has been complaining about her ceiling chandeliers shaking too much. She is afraid they are going to drop on her head. Mama says the neighbor downstairs is a troublemaker. How much can three little children shake the floor while jumping? The neighbor doesn't understand because she is childless.

I love Sunday mornings when my brothers and I are allowed to get in bed with our parents. My favorite game is putting my finger on Papa's lips, and then pulling it off before he bites my finger. But he never bites me for real, and if he does he rolls his lips over his teeth so he doesn't hurt me. I also like to be tickled and jump up and down on their bed.

Mama tried making some artwork for sale. She made a collage out of different paper prints and glued the pieces to pottery. Papa, who is a perfectionist, felt it was very poor work and stated that no one — in his right mind — would buy it.

If Mama finds out that I have not gone to the bathroom for more than two days, I get an enema. I don't like enemas; I hate baring my bottom to the whole world to see and lying down on her lap so she can give me an enema. It's always done in the room next to the bathroom or in the kitchen so we can get to the toilet as fast as we can. It only feels good when it all comes out. Seems like once a week whether we like it or not my brothers and I get enemas.

Mama is fulfilling her desire of becoming a medical doctor like her brother and cousins. Her first love was to conduct an orchestra. She had been given a scholarship to go to England to study and become a *maestro*, but her parents loved her too much to lose her into the big sinful and cruel world where anything bad can happen when you are an innocent beautiful young girl living far away from home without adult supervision. Her parents would not allow that to happen. In those days, women left the parent's house for two reasons only, to get married or to become a nun. Being a concert pianist and getting her musical degree in Lisbon, not far from the family, was fine as long as she was home before it got dark outside.

Mama's career now is being a mommy to my brothers and I, but that is not good enough for her. She is our doctor too; after all, being a doctor is just a minor technical term having to do with some schooling and a medical degree. Her brother Augusto and cousins had done that, but as a member of the family she feels she is entitled to a certain degree of respect, which dictates she knows just about as much as they do, except for surgery of course. It's not only Mama that acts like a doctor, Aunt Heydee also knows a lot about drugs and dispenses them as she gets them from our medical family members as needed for colds, bellyaches, fevers, anemia, headaches, nerves, and so on. For whatever ails anyone, there's always something to take from Aunt Heydee or Mama's small pharmacy. Each owns a few shoeboxes full of medicine. Besides giving penicillin shots and enemas, Mama is also good at using the suction glasses on anyone that has a chest cold, pleurisy or backache, this treatment also helps to clear lung congestion. Mama lights up a match and throws it into a small glass that has a little piece of cotton inside, and then turns the glass over on the area being treated, most of the time it's the back. Suction starts and it's fun to watch the skin lifting up like a bubble and getting red. This treatment comes from the medical doctors in China, and somehow has been passed onto the women's side of Grandma's family from generation to generation. It's that easy to learn.

Winter of 1950

Mama made me a homemade costume for *Carnaval.* We can't afford to rent one. She bought a few yards of colorful starched cotton cloth with a pattern of colorful roses, which I wore on top of my regular warm winter flannel green dress, and she made a red apron and a flowery scarf to match the skirt. When no one is looking I like rubbing my nose on the vibrant colorful skirt and smelling the starched new material. I never had anything so crispy and fresh in my life, except for the organza white dress I used to have when I was one year old. Mama painted my face with lots of makeup and she even drew a nice size black mole on my left cheek, just like she uses when she gets all dressed up to go out with Papa. As a final touch she stuck a big plastic flower on my black fuzzy hat. I looked like a real Portuguese country girl. I really loved having Mama so close to me, combing my hair and trying to make me pretty. She promised that next year when she wins the lottery she would rent a real professional outfit for me to wear at *Carnaval.* She said I can be a princess, but I told her that I'd rather dress up as a pirate.

Spring of 1950

The porter and some of the neighbors are plotting to evict us from our apartment. Mama is very upset about this. It's not our fault that we are poor and don't have electricity in the house. We use candles at night for dinner and then we go to bed. She keeps pointing her finger above her head as if towards some invisible power above as she says that God is good and He will protect us from our enemies and their evil ways.

It just happened that while having lunch, Mama got a cod fish bone stuck in her throat. We were on our way to the emergency squad, which is now appropriately situated at the corner of our street, and she was running down our apartment house steps, holding her throat while gasping for air when she saw the porter downstairs.

He asked her what was wrong and Mama immediately in an act of desperation put her whole hand in her mouth and down her throat and removed the fish bone herself, saying right after, "Nothing is wrong *senhor* Rodrigues."

That was a very heroic moment for Mama who wouldn't give the porter the satisfaction of seeing her choke to death.

Mama bragged to Papa that evening about her quick response to the mean and nasty porter and Papa went on and on about how dumb the whole thing was. He had never heard of anyone choking on a fish bone, at least not so often like Mama does.

"It's all a matter of upbringing," he said in his heavy German accent. As a child he had won an award for best manners at the table and being able to eat a fish to such perfection that only the skeleton was left on the plate with every single bone in its proper position. He was only eight years old, but that's how it is in Germany, everyone learns at a very young age how to eat fish.

I had a horrible birthday! Someone told Mama that the dandelions growing in our yard, which is nothing but weeds, could be converted into delicious nourishing soup.

I saw her picking them up and boiling them with old dark moldy bread. I would so much rather have rice pudding. The smell from the soup was a sour green spoiled smell. It was enough to make anyone puke, which I did, but that didn't stop her from making me eat it. I got hit with the wooden spoon over the head over and over again.

"If you don't eat, you are going to die from starvation," she said.

Then, as if that was not enough torture she gave me her birthday gift. A wool dress she made out of every leftover wool piece she had collected through the years. It was too big. It was lumpy where the strings were tied with one another. It had millions of colors and it made me itch. I didn't want to wear it. It was a warm day. But she made me not only put it on but took me into the backyard and forced me to sit down on the old wooden garden chair and smile as if I was happy to the camera. Her brother Augusto loaned her his camera because he was too busy to see me on my birthday.

Summer of 1950

Luisa, the little girl that lives in our building on the second floor, was playing in her yard, and when she saw me leaning over her fence, she invited me to come in and play with her. We sat on the grass by the peppermint bushes and she started to put peppermint leaves inside her vagina.

She wanted me to do it too but I told her that I couldn't because I was afraid that the leaves might have gross little bugs on them, and besides, I'd rather use peppermint in tea with a lemon twist, like Grandma Rica drinks. She asked me not to tell anyone or she would get into trouble. I have not seen her since that day when we played in her backyard. Maybe her Mama saw everything from their window and now Luisa is not allowed out anymore. It's too bad, because I would like to have a friend to play with. I am not allowed to go upstairs to find out what happened to Luisa. Mama said they moved away.

I went to her backyard this morning and found the green door to her garden locked from the inside.

Mama was telling us a story today about the grandmother that came to live with her daughter and was given a metal cup and a metal dish to use during her meals.

When the granddaughter saw that, she asked her mother, "Why doesn't grandma eat from china dishes and crystal glasses, like us?"

"Because she is old and weak. If she uses the expensive dinnerware she might drop it and break it."

And the little girl said, "I understand. That is a very good reason. I promise when you get to be old like grandma, I will also give you unbreakable metal dinnerware to eat from."

Her mother realized that she was wrong and, hoping her daughter would not do that to her when she got old, she gave her mother the best of chinaware and also the most beautiful crystal glass to drink water from. I love stories. I know this is a corny one, and Mama probably made it up, but I like when Mama talks to us.

Autumn of 1950

I am in first grade and I don't like school; the teachers are always hitting my hands with a wooden ruler. There are other girls like me that get punished. I just hope I will never have to be punished like some girls that are forced to wear donkey ears cut out of newspapers and wear them like a hat, and then as if that's not degrading enough they have to sit in a chair outside on the veranda, facing the street so that people going by can look at them and laugh. My wrists got so sore this week from getting hit with the ruler that Mama felt sorry for me and wrapped both my wrists in bandages and sent me back the next day with a medical excuse note from Uncle Augusto, stating that my wrists are very weak and I'm not to get hit or my wrists will break. Now they hit me over the head, and my head is lumpy. I hate school.

Grandma gave us some of her old furniture and now we have a china cabinet and a nice big table back in the empty room where we used to have our meals. I didn't mind eating in the kitchen, I thought it was fun, but in the winter it is too cold. Mama said we would return to having our meals in the kitchen when it's summertime so that we can stay cool.

Winter of 1951

Wintertime is museum time. I love museums and the mystery of ages that come with them. Times of long ago still breathing by our side, like friendly ghosts from the past. I have never seen a ghost but just about everybody else has. The idea really scares me. I believe that dead people should be visiting only other dead people. We went to the Monastery dos Jerónimos, this weekend. It was a family group outing with Mama, Aunt Heydee, my brothers and Maria, the part-time maid who knows how to keep my brothers and I from running around and getting into mischief. We entered a huge badly lit room built hundreds of years ago with high vaulted stonewalls. The air felt stagnant and as old as the walls around.

I heard Aunt Heydee saying, "Look it's the tomb of the Unknown Soldier, everybody take a look."

Not me, why would I want to see a dead soldier? Guts coming out, eyes bugged out with the worms eating his flesh, the bony hands stretched out seeking someone's help as if screaming for help. He had to be screaming even if we heard no sound. When you no longer have a throat and all the bones are just rotting away and you have been locked up inside the coffin for centuries, only silence can be heard. But is he really silent or just waiting? Is the coffin open or closed? And if it's closed, does he still have enough power left to open it, get out and grab us?

My two brothers ran towards the tomb and I ran towards the exit. Maria grabbed me by the waist holding me under her arm, and started to walk to the tomb, saying, "There is nothing to be afraid of, now take a look!"

I was screaming and had my eyes tightly squeezed shut. "No," I screamed, "I don't want to look, put me down!!!"

She stopped walking and I could tell she was by the tomb. She put me down. I opened my eyes just a little to see where I was and I walked away from the stone coffin very carefully not to look in that direction. Everybody was laughing and making fun of me, calling me chicken. But I didn't care; I know that I am not a chicken, because if I were one, I would lay eggs.

~ *Chapter Three* ~

The Learning Years

1951-1955

Spring of 1951

A lot of commotion went on in our apartment building one evening. We were getting ready to go to bed when the maid from the third floor came down to invite my brothers and me to a special event. It was very crowded and many other children that I had never met were already seated on their sunroom's floor. The father of the birthday boy closed the curtains and turned off all the lights to make the room dark, then he cranked the handle on the movie machine and the light coming from the machine projected on the wall a real American movie with Cowboys and Indians. There was no sound coming from the wall, like in the movie theatre, but we knew from the actor's expressions and movements what was happening, and at the end of the movie, the handsome cowboy kissed the horse's nose and they both walked away into the sunset. It was a very emotional moment. We applauded and screamed, so happy we were, and we all asked to see the movie one more time since it was very good but only lasted a few minutes. The boy's father re-winded the film in the machine and ran it one more time while we all sat quietly in complete amazement. This is what I call an incredible invention. I can't believe what I saw, and it was so exciting. Movies at home!

Mama was out with José. She is always taking him to the doctors to see if they have a drug to cure him. Max-Leão and I were left alone at home. We started looking around inside the closets for something to play with. We found some jars made of transparent glass with engraved flowers and pelicans; we could tell they were very special jars because they were hidden way in the back of the closet and out of sight. We found a bottle almost half-filled with a clear liquid and a white tree branch inside of it. The label read, *Anise*. We sniffed the *anise* and it smelled real good, so we took a turn each having a mouth full of the sweet liquor inside. When we finished drinking we went to the kitchen and got a knife to yank out the small pieces of sugar branches from inside the bottle, which tasted like the best candy we'd ever had. Just then, Mama came home and there she found us sitting on the floor holding the empty bottle. She was very upset. We had just drunk and eaten the only *anise* left in the house, but since the valuable jars were not damaged she didn't even hit us, saying, "Well, I don't have to worry about you two anymore, because the last drop of alcohol in this house is now gone."

Nothing special happens anymore on my birthday. The good old days are gone. I hinted to Mama that I wish I had a birthday cake. She got me a cupcake and put a candle in the middle of it. I acted like I was very happy about it. I didn't want to hurt her feelings over the clothes she made for me, but she could tell that I was not happy. I have to learn to hide my feelings better, otherwise I will have to explain why I am sad, and then I feel guilty.

I have to remember that there are other kids in a worse situation than me, even though Mama keeps saying that I was born with a silver spoon in my mouth. Our last dainty German gold glass with an engraved lady's face on it is gone again. Mama told me it is in the pawnshop. Mama has been cooking and cleaning. I have not seen Maria, the maid. Obviously Papa is not selling enough magazines to pay the rent or to buy food either. I understand what's going on without anyone telling me. We communicate in a silent language.

It was José's birthday this weekend and Papa and Mama played with us. Papa told us he was going to take us all on a fun trip. The room where Max-Leão and I used to sleep is now empty. We both sleep in what used to be the guestroom. José continues to sleep in our parent's room in case they have to rush him to the hospital during the night because of an asthma attack.

Papa made a big secret over our mystery trip. It was going to happen inside the empty room and only one of us could go in at a time, with Papa as the leader and Mama as his assistant. José was the first one to go in with his eyes covered by a scarf. The door closed behind them. Max-Leão and I sat on the hallway floor waiting nervously for our turn. José came out still with his eyes covered and laughing. We were no longer scared. I was next. Mama put the scarf over my eyes and Papa told me I was not allowed to peek, as he held my hand. And into the room we went. It was very windy.

"Feel the wind blowing?" I heard Papa saying, "It's a storm!" I wondered where the wind could be coming from since it is a room without a window.

"Yes, yes," I said a bit skeptical but very happy and excited.

"Soon, it's going to start raining," said Mama, adding, "Feel the rain, on your face?"

"Yes, yes," I said once again wondering how the weather elements had got inside of an empty apartment room. "It's wonderful," I said, deciding to just enjoy it and go with it.

"Here is an umbrella, hold onto it," said Papa, as he put an umbrella in my hand.

"Verónica, put it over your head, it's raining in the garden." I heard Mama's voice.

The Magic Room.

"The sun just came out, give me the umbrella back." I heard Papa as he added, "Hold my hand and let's go up the steps climbing high towards the moon. Be careful. Don't trip. Wow, you have reached the moon, now jump off, down to earth, it's okay I'll catch you."

I was a little scared about that, but since it was all imagination nothing could hurt me. I could tell that Papa was holding me in the air. I moved my arms like the wings of a bird, and I had to laugh as I landed softly on the ground. What a trip! I found myself out of the room.

"Okay, now its Max-Leão's turn," and Papa took off the scarf covering my eyes. "You can watch how this is done, if you promise to be very quiet," he said.

I promised to be good and not to say a word. Once again I entered the magic room. This time my eyes were wide open and looking for answers. The room was empty except for a wooden ladder in the middle of the room. Next to it was our old metal garden water can, Papa's rusty, green fan and his big black umbrella. I had to smile, I was so happy to find that the mind can create anything with the help of sound, a touch, and the love of my parents. For a few moments, there was magic.

After dinner I mentioned how I would love to go on an imaginary trip again. But Mama said it would be a while before they had the time to do that with us again. Papa went on to tell us about his home in Berlin, Germany and how his parents used to play games like these with him and his two sisters, Ilse and Friedel, when they were about our age. They even had a mini-theater in one of the rooms of their house where they used to put on hand puppet shows for their parents, family, and friends. In those days Papa's voice was very weak and he could barely speak as a child. He had been born with a defective throat and it wasn't until he was eight years old that his parents took him to a throat specialist who knew how to fix that kind of problem. So until he was eight years old he was only able to play the piano but he couldn't sing or act a part in the puppet shows. This is the reason why Papa even today won't talk on the phone, he is very conscious of his voice not having a normal pitch and a few times he was mistaken as woman's voice on the phone. He feels very embarrassed about it. He had to struggle with this handicap all his life, and if it hadn't been for that surgeon who did the surgery Papa would be a mute.

Papa's parents were very rich and their house was on the same street as other very important people in the government. Across the street from his house lived the chancellor of Berlin. Papa still remembers the chancellor because he always smiled and waived at him from inside his golden coach pulled by horses. On weekends Papa's parents gave parties and they had famous pianists and opera singers hired to entertain their guests. I love hearing stories of the past because I get to know that my parents were also children sometime ago, just like my brothers and I.

Summer of 1951

It has been very, very hot in the last few days. My two brothers and I are allowed to take our clothes off and bathe inside the washbasin in the sunroom. This must be the way it feels like to be in a swimming pool, cool and not scary like the ocean with big waves.

Max-Leão and I talked about having a real swimming pool built in our yard. How difficult can it be? We only need to take out the *nespra* tree and dig a square hole in the ground and fill it with water. He is going to talk to Mama and Papa and see if he can convince them this is a great idea. They should be very happy that we are willing to do all the digging; they just have to supply us with water.

We were coming back from our evening stroll to the park down the street and Mama was pushing José in his stroller when suddenly a nice lady at a window turned out to be Encarnação, a friend of Mama from the old days when they both were students at the Music Conservatory. It just happened that she lives down the street from our house. All these years and they didn't even know. Encarnação happened to be looking out at her windowsill, enjoying the fresh air, when we were going by. She doesn't wear makeup. Her hair is not colored like Mama's either; instead it has shades of gray. She is built like a workingwoman, stocky, she is as big as Mama. I liked Encarnação because she seemed kind and smiled a lot. They reminisced for a while about their younger days in school. She is a widow and has two grown-up daughters and a sixteen-year-old son. They exchanged phone numbers.

When Papa got home a few days ago Mama told him about Max-Leão and I fighting with each other, and that we should get punished. Papa told us both to go to our backyard and get a thick, large stick for him to hit us with.

We looked around the yard and when I picked up a stick Max-Leão said, "Are you crazy, he's going to kill us with a stick that size, let's give him this little one. We'll tell him this was the biggest one we found."

Together we carried a little dried-up twig branch from our backyard and we carried it as if it was big and heavy.

"I asked for a big wooden stick to beat you with and this is all you can find?" Papa was obviously not falling for Max-Leão's great idea.

I almost died when I heard Max-Leão saying with an innocent look on his face, "This was the biggest stick we could find."

I nodded my head in agreement.

The fear in our eyes and the size of the stick we brought to Papa mellowed his anger.

He laughed and said, "Okay, I'll forgive you both this time, but next time you are bad I won't be so nice, you will get double the punishment."

Max-Leão and I talked about this experience and we are going to try the same trick the next time. We are so smart!

Autumn of 1951

I miss the Sunday mornings when my brothers and I used to lay down with our parents, playing and talking about silly things that made us all laugh. They say we are too old for that now.

I got to impress them both this morning with the unique sounds I can make with my tongue. They were both seated on the veranda, enjoying their Sunday morning, and I said, "Would you like to hear me make the sound of a horse?" And I went right on clicking my tongue against the roof of my mouth, *click, clunk, click, clunk*. They were both very impressed with my talent and they both were laughing and feeling happy. I love seeing my parents seated together and laughing. I also showed them how I can feel my mouth with air and by parting my lips just a little I can make funny sounds when I press both my index fingers against each of my cheeks. They love me.

I got into big trouble today for no reason. Max-Leão and I were helping José, who is a lot smaller than us, because he is only three years old, to climb out of the front window in our bedroom facing the street and to get on his knees between two of the empty potholders so that he could throw the dirt on the people walking on the street. We simply wanted to have some fun with the flowerless clay pots. A long time ago there had been six flowered plants growing, but with time the plants had died and all that was left was dried up dirt inside the clay pots. It was all going fine, Max-Leão and I were holding José by the suspenders and we were having a good time laughing when the neighbor across the street started screaming that José was going to fall off the windowsill. José got scared with her screams and dropped one of the clay pots, missing some people walking underneath our window. It was an accident. They called the police and the neighbor said we were a hazard in the neighborhood and that our parents had to punish us. Max-Leão and I were accused of possibly killing José had he fallen off the window with the

Just Having Fun.

clay pot. I tried to explain that I was holding him by the suspenders the whole time and he was perfectly safe that way. I promised that I would never again throw dirt into the street. It didn't do any good, we got punished and once again Max-Leão and I couldn't sit for days. José didn't get punished because he is too sickly to suffer a beating.

Mama says that I did very well in school last year and this year it will be easier. It's not true. The teachers are just as mean as the others, and I am confused about what they say and what they write on the blackboard. I still don't understand anything, and math is the worst ever except for the tables of multiplication, I memorized those out of desperation. If I don't I will get donkey ears.

My school is only a couple of blocks down the hill from where we live, on a long and steep street called Calçada de Arroios. Last year I was chaperoned to school but now that I am older I am allowed to go by myself, as long as I don't talk to or go with any strangers. I always rush down the hill to get to school on time and I like running across the little round park that looks like an island with three palm trees, lots of flowers, and two wooden benches for the older folks.

The street going down from the corner of our house is made with cobblestones just like all the streets in Lisbon, but it is very steep. I can run up with no problem, but if I ran down carelessly and without looking down for holes and bumps on the sidewalk I will hit the tip of my shoe on something and fall.

I have bruised knees and elbows from falling several times going down the Calçada de Arroios. The reason the streets are so steep is because of earthquakes. When the ground moves it produces hills filled with bodies and houses that fall trapped under the ground. The big one in 1755 literally destroyed Lisbon. It all happened in the middle of the day, about lunchtime. All the men working in the factories making bricks got instantly buried, that's why we always say, when somebody dies, "They went to make bricks."

Aunt Heydee rarely falls, but she told me that she does get her high heels sometimes stuck between the cobblestones and a few times twisted her ankles, but that's it. She always wears very, very high heels because she is too short without them and men like tall women.

When school is over for the day, I love taking my time to get home. I like getting underneath the water drains coming down from the buildings and getting soaked to the skin, I love hearing the sound and the feel of my shoes squeaking as I walk. Rain is a lot of fun. I love rain because it's just like taking a shower. We still don't have a bathtub; maybe someday we will have a tub, when we are rich again.

Whatever I get in life that is good, I am very thankful for it. And I am very thankful for Encarnação, my mother's friend. She is my best friend. I go to her house every time I can. She lets me help her to make cakes and chocolate cookies and today she braided my hair and said that I was pretty, and that she wished I were her daughter. When I got home, Mama saw my new hairdo and was very upset. I am not to have anybody touch my hair. If I want to look like an old lady with the hair up, she is not going to allow it. She took the pins out of my hair, combed and parted it to the side straight, the way she likes it. I am afraid Mama will stop me from going to visit Encarnação, so when I come home, I remove the hairpins off my hair before I climb the steps to our house. I don't really mind doing that, since the tight hair pulled back by the pins gives me a headache. Encarnação is happy that my hair is pulled back and I look neat and pretty when I spend the day with her. Mama is happy to see me ugly with my hair pulled down straight to the side. How easy it is to make everybody happy.

Max-Leão and I like to sit at the veranda of our parent's bedroom watching the people and cars go by. He can always tell what brand and year a car is, even from far away, even before it reaches our street. He is very smart. To me all the cars look the same except for different colors. Our favorite

---

pastime game is watching the funeral processions. We count how many cars are following the black decorated carriage with heavy chunky golden angels. If it is a long procession that means the person that died was very popular. The carriage is usually pulled by four, sometimes six horses, which are dressed in colorful gold mountings and decorated with lots of flowers. The flowers are all over the horses and on the roof of the carriage. Two men dressed in black with matching black top hats sit on a stool pulling the reins that control the horses to strut at a steady pace. I don't understand why they have to kill so many flowers when someone dies.

Chest X-rays are now mandatory at school. A lot of children were found to have tuberculosis and they were not allowed to return to school. My chest X-ray shows that I have a scar in the left lung due to early tuberculosis. I am very lucky that I didn't die. I had TB when I was a lot younger and no one even knew it. This means that I am a weakling and I will always be sickly and can never do hard work. I will always have to bundle up in the winter and if I don't eat more bread and soup I will die. Mama took me to see our cousin Salomão, who is a heart specialist, and he took another X-ray of my chest in his office to confirm that my TB is not active. I don't know why, but I don't like him or his office.

Encarnação has an adopted niece. Her name is Maria Leonor. She is my own age and I am allowed to visit and play with her at Encarnação's house. I would love to look like her with blonde hair, blue eyes, and very white, almost see-through skin. She is very pretty. She came over to our house once but was not allowed in. It is something to do with my two brothers; one of them might like her as a future girlfriend and that can never happen, as she is of a different religion.

The last time I saw Maria Leonor was last summer; she came over to our house and we both sat on the black metal steps in back of our house eating cherries from a straw basket she had brought with her. We hung the cherries on our earlobes like earrings and talked and laughed. Maria

Leonor is very lucky; she gets to visit Encarnação a lot more than me. I heard that Maria Leonor has been sick for the last few months. Nobody knows what's wrong.

On weekends I visit Encarnação, and I spend a lot of time in her deceased husband's study. She left everything just the way he used to have it before he died. I love looking into the African books, with pictures of people with black skin and big lips stretched by dishes inside the inner lips. She told me these books are from the time when her dead husband was the ambassador from Portugal to Angola and she lived in Africa with him. She actually saw wild animals in the jungle, and the people were black and walked naked because they were very poor savages. I don't blame them; it looks like it's very, very hot in Africa. Their skin is probably black from being burned in the hot sun everyday.

I have become a reader; I love reading books on adventure and other countries far away. *Gulliver's Travels* and *The Swiss Family Robinson* are both my favorites, and I have read them over and over again. Someday I will travel to faraway countries and write about my adventures.

Mama is always happy to send me to Encarnação's house after school. Encarnação loves me. She feeds me and keeps me warm. I love her kitchen with the big glass windows that open to her garden. The sunshine brightens the kitchen, which is always warm and cheery. The smells of a Portuguese house are alive in her house, alive with the soft scent of olive oil pouring out from one of the large wooden barrels into the glass containers in the pantry next to the kitchen. The fresh batter for cakes and cookies is even tastier than when cooked. I love raw batter. I like to help beating the eggs and peeling the almond skins after they are scalded and then crunching them, and I also like to help ground the fresh meat with the added herbs and moist bread soaked in milk. Encarnação has two maids always cooking when she is getting ready to entertain. She has a large family, but she still has room for me. She is always home, and she loves her family and all her friends.

Over the weekend Mama had to call Uncle Augusto because I was having a stomach ache and she thought I might need surgery. I was scared. Uncle Augusto couldn't come to see me because he was too busy. He told Mama over the phone to put ice on my abdomen and if it went away it was not appendicitis. It went away, thank God!

Papa scares me when he has a temper attack. Last night Grandma Rica and Aunt Heydee came over for dinner. Aunt Heydee was telling Papa that Germans are bad people, that they are all Nazis.

Papa said that the German people are good people and they don't have anything to do with the Nazi philosophy.

But Aunt Heydee insisted that if he was defending the Germans he was a Nazi too.

Papa got very angry and yelled at her, "I am German, and proud of it." He then picked up the white table cloth with the food and dishes and pulled everything off the table — like you see professional magicians doing — except that when Papa pulled the table cloth, everything went flying, including the food on the dishes and serving platters and the glasses with milk and water splattering all over the floor along with the crashed dishes. Mama and Grandma Rica were crying and my brothers and I were sent to bed right after that.

This has happened before, where Aunt Heydee and Papa are having a dispute over world politics, and she drives him crazy with anger. Something always goes flying into the air. Mama says this whole thing has stemmed out of Papa having to wait ten years before Aunt Heydee said, "Ok, you can marry my sister."

He will never forgive her for that.

In the summer of 1933, Papa came to Portugal for the first time. His job until then was managing the production of hand made embroidery and lace in the Portuguese Islands of Azores and then exporting it to Germany where his parents

Papa's Bad Temper.

had a few lace factories. He was visiting Portugal as a possible country to seek refuge, after a German Navy Admiral visiting the Island of Azores where my father was staying, confided in him that since Hitler had been made Chancellor of Germany in the beginning of that year, the world was never going to be the same. As a Jew he should never return to Germany and if anything he should send word to his family to get the heck out as soon as possible and as far away as they could. Papa sent the information to his family and was waiting to hear from them. While in Lisbon he was invited to a private party, and that was where he met Mama for the first time. Papa was playing the piano when Mama and her sisters walked in. Papa saw her as the most beautiful woman he had ever seen. She was wearing a white dress and a tan that made her skin glow. Mama and her two sisters Heydee and Ligia had spent the day at the beach. Mama had dark brown hair that was naturally curly and worn down to her shoulders with a face that melted him away; she looked like a goddess, he said. She sat next to him and started playing the piano along with him. He couldn't help but falling in love with her right then and there. The problem was that he was a foreigner and without a job.

When he asked Aunt Heydee for Mama's hand in marriage, she told him, "Come back only when you have your own business, a secure paying job, here in Portugal, so that my sister doesn't have to go away, like my other sister Nelly."

Ten years later he did return, as co-owner of a German restaurant in downtown Lisbon, and Aunt Heydee gave my future parents her blessing.

Winter of 1952

When someone can take me to Grandma Rica's house, it's usually on weekends. When she baby-sits for my brothers and me, she teaches us French and math. Her house is on the other side of the city and we are not allowed to walk that far by ourselves. I see Encarnação a lot more often because she lives closer to our house. She has been teaching me to do crochet, but Mama found out about it and told me that only old ladies do that kind of work, and besides it's not good for the eyes to strain them with such fine needlework. I am not allowed to crochet anymore. Mama showed me how to knit instead, which in reality is a lot easier because the needles are huge, and the final product gets done faster. I am making a long wool scarf with Mama and a dainty crochet piece at Encarnação's house, but that is a secret between Encarnação and me.

Wintertime with Encarnação is always wonderful! We both sit in the living room, where she has a small round tea table with a charcoal fire underneath it. This is the only heating system in the whole house. But it's more than what we have for we don't have anything to heat our house with. When her daughters are visiting her, we all sit around her tea table, keeping our feet warm, and we eat roasted chestnuts and lots of hot milk with a dash of coffee.

Encarnacão's son Eduardo is very nice to me and he lets me play with his toy airplanes. He told me that someday he is going to be a pilot. His two sisters are beyond their teens. They are grownups. Bonéca the youngest is going to be a flight attendant, because she is very beautiful, she looks like a model. Her sister Annette is not pretty, but she is getting married in a few months. Mama hired her to tutor me in math. I don't like Encarnacão's daughters. Bonéca was making fun of the way I dress. I happen to agree, but that doesn't give her the right to pick me up in the air and lift my skirt to show my underwear to the maids in the kitchen. They made fun of me and laughed loudly at my colorful underwear. If Encarnação had found out she would have punished her, I am sure of that. I will never talk to Bonéca again and I will hate her forever. She may be very beautiful on the outside, but inside she is an ugly monster.

I have watched Mama making my underwear. She cuts two squares out of two pieces of very colorful cotton and then she cuts a V-shape at the bottom to make way to the legs, and sows it that way. After that she inserts a drawstring at the waist to tie it up — only, when she has elastic band available she uses that instead. Because she is trying to make them last a few years they are usually too big for me so I have to roll them around my waist which makes me look fat and square. Someday I will have normal underwear, but right now we can't afford extra frivolous stuff.

Annette never smiles, and treats me like a child that is brothering her. She uses a pencil for torturing me and every time I make a mistake in math she hits my knuckles with it. I feel sorry for her future children, if she is going to teach them math, they will wind up with bumpy ugly knuckles, probably to match their ugly faces, like their mother. Encarnação's daughters are nasty. I went home and cried this afternoon. I wasn't going to cry in front of Annette no matter how much it hurt. Mama saw my red knuckles and I'm now without a math tutor.

I like my friends at school, but not the curriculum. I am a terrible student. I don't understand what the teacher says, it all sounds like *jibber, jibber, jibber*. I get bored and I try very hard to stay awake in class by chewing on pencils and sticking the tip between my gums. The school building is very old and smells of ink, rotten wood and books. The classes are very large and overcrowded.

Mama told a fib to the teacher so she would put me in the front row. Mama told the teacher that I don't see or hear too well, and unless I'm sitting up front I will learn absolutely nothing.

Across the little round park in front of our school, there's a tall white church. I like to go inside once in awhile just to see why everybody likes to go in. They say God lives there but all I see are gray stone tombs, stone angels, and saints surrounded by candles. It's hard to see and breathe inside the old church. I feel much happier when I come out to the fresh air outside. I doubt that God lives inside that church; if I was God, I would not want to live in a dreary place like that.

Back and forth from school I enjoy walking into the shops and listening to the shop vendors and their customers. I like wandering in and out of their shops and looking around to see what kind of merchandise they have and what's new. Across the street from our house, the cranky lady in the cave below the first floor has no shop, just a window that opens to the street where her female clients drop off sheer silk stockings to be mended. Sometimes Mama sends me over there with a couple of her silk stockings to be fixed; it's cheaper to fix them than to buy a new pair. The stocking lady never talks to me except for giving me a scribbled receipt and saying, "You can pick them up next week." And then she closes her little window.

Around the corner, the shoemaker also has a window on the ground floor, leveled to the sidewalk but he keeps it opened and he always welcomes an exchange of small talk, and has told me his dream. Someday soon he will be going to North America with his wife and children. He has put in all the necessary papers with our government, and now he has to wait patiently.

Down the street from him there's a big grocery store, Mr. António is the owner and he is always there, standing by the door of his establishment. He runs a fully packed grocery store with lots of burlap bags full of potatoes and grains and legumes and all kinds of dry goods. It's very difficult to see clearly indoors because Mr. António never turns on the lights inside the store. It seems to me that he is trying to save electricity, or he belongs to the bat family. I don't have the courage to say anything, but I believe that I could make his grocery store a lot more attractive by having everything more neatly organized. Maybe because it's hard to see inside the shop, that's why it's so crammed full and cluttered. I don't know how he finds anything in the dark. He never smiles and doesn't seem happy. Mama buys all our dry groceries from him, she calls him on the phone and then his grocery boy delivers the groceries to our house.

The bakery on the corner only makes bread, and everything is covered with white flour, including the floors, walls and the workers. I would not want to hug a baker. It has got to be the whitest bakery I have ever seen. In the wintertime, it is the place where I take our dinner once in awhile to be baked. For a couple of *escudos* they let us use their oven, and we use it when Mama makes our favorite meal, *Empadão de carne*. I love *Empadão de carne*, it is really yummy, and I specially love the salty oily black olives studded into the golden mashed potatoes on top of the ground meat.

The storekeeper in the gift shop is always telling me to either buy something or get out. She must be afraid I will hear some top-secret gossip news about someone in the neighborhood. This is the gossip shop; the women in the area seem to gather there to talk about everybody else. Some women are dressed in black from head to toe, which means they lost a family member. This goes on for a year, even two years, but if one of them is dressed in black year after year it means she lost her husband or son possibly to the sea or maybe a car accident. In Portugal when there's a car accident, most of the time someone dies because most drivers are compelled to drive too fast and don't like to follow the laws of the road. Like frustrated bull fighters, they see the car coming towards them as the bull and themselves as the *matador*.

The manual workers favorite places for lunch are the two taverns that are between our house and my school down the street. There are also the regulars who spend the day drinking and pass the time talking to each other and socializing. I like walking into the taverns making believe that I'm looking for somebody and then walk out, hitting the beaded curtains on purpose with my shoulders so that they make a rattling noise as they swing into each other. I would like to know what men talk about in these dark taverns and why they drink so much. They probably like the smell of wine mixed with fish stew and olives, or maybe they tell stories of pirates and islands far away and treasures hidden inside some caves by the shore. It's even darker in these taverns than at Mr. António's grocery store, possibly because both taverns are narrow and deep and their doorways are covered by long wood-beaded curtains that block the sun from coming in, like the beaded curtains found at the meat market's doorway. During the summer these curtains are supposed to keep the flies from entering. I like feeling the beads on my face and body when I walk in and out that is, if the owner of the establishment doesn't get annoyed and throw me out. I keep going around and around, under the beaded curtains until they tangle around me, then I listen to the rattling sound they make against each other as they slide back down to their original place. Most of the men inside are old and cranky and they get annoyed with me, calling me a child and telling me to get lost. They have no humor. They were born only to drink. Both taverns' walls are covered by large wine wood barrels stacked one on top of the other to make more room for customers to walk in, but that also obstructs the light from entering the already small narrow establishments.

I still don't like school; I am barely passing the tests. We all sit in our own designated wood chair attached to a desk. There's a small round hole to the right of the desktop where we keep the glass inkwell along with the blotter and a long wooden fountain pen. We have to use a lot of care not to damage its delicate metal tip. We also use pencils, and writing with ink is a lot more fun, but if we are not careful and put too much ink in the tip of the pen it's a real mess when it drips on the paper. Not to mention the teacher getting angry. I have gotten very good at using the blotter to go over the wet writing. I like the smell of ink. Next to my desk there's another girl and when she writes with her left hand the teacher yells at her and says she is possessed by the devil. She gets hit a lot over the knuckles and over her head with the wooden ruler. The teacher won't allow her to write with her left hand.

I am very lucky that I am right handed but I have to wear wristbands to protect my weak wrists or I'll get hit with the ruler until they are red and swollen.

Spring of 1952

I like biting my fingernails as much as Max-Leão. I stopped biting my toenails a few years ago, when my feet would no longer come up to my mouth that easily. Max-Leão and I were taken to the kitchen to be punished for our bad habit. José doesn't bite his nails. He doesn't have any bad habits. He suffers from asthma. I was scared, I thought that we were going to get beat up with some kitchen utensil. Aunt Heydee, Papa, and Mama were working together and Aunt Heydee showed her concern by stating that only low-class uneducated people have such a nasty habit. Mama held Max-Leão's hands and started rubbing a hot pepper on his fingernails.

"That will burn your lips every time you put your fingers to your mouth," said Josefina, the part-time maid with a wacky look in her eyes. Ironically, she also bites her own fingernails but blames it on doing dishes and laundry.

Then the unthinkable happened: Max-Leão immediately put his fingers in his mouth and said in amazement, "Wow, this stuff is really good."

When I heard that, I requested some peppers too.

Papa said, "This is not working out. Maybe soap is better. How about using soap for Verónica."

But Mama didn't agree, "Verónica loves soap, she will be sucking at her fingernails even more."

Giving up on us, they told us that every time they see us with our hands in our mouth we are getting slapped right across the face. This is so unfair; I don't see what's wrong with biting my nails. I don't swallow them I spit them out. Max-Leão and I decided that we would bite our nails when we are alone in our beds.

Max-Leão and I sometimes get into fights against other kids in our neighborhood. It happens mostly at the parks where we play or on the way home from the parks. A few times we had to fight with our fists. Sometimes I go home with a bloody nose. The neighbor boys are a bunch of bullies. Mama says I am more like a tomboy than a girl, but that's not true, I am only defending myself.

I no longer go around pushing other kid's faces into the water fountain. One of the other boys thought it was funny to do it back at me and I didn't like the way it felt when my mouth hit the metal faucet and I got a bloody lip. I have noticed that whatever I do to someone, I get the same back; so I have to be careful not to hurt anybody anymore, unless I am defending my life and my brothers are with me.

Our garden has long been gone. The walls around it are easy to peel and inside the pitted holes are the homes for the worms and the salamanders. When I am bored I peel the chipped paint from the backyard's wall, looking to find the worms that, upon being touched, curl up for protection. Some people call them pill bugs or sow bugs. I call them roly-polys. They have very strong muscles, and it's hard to open them again, so I set them up on top of the wall and with a flick of my fingers, I see how far I can fling them into the distance.

The green wooden door has lost its color and the hinges are corroded by the weather and neglect. To enter our backyard the door has to be lifted and then dropped, otherwise it will stay up in the air. Our garden is just an arid area of dirt with a few stalks of artichokes, which I eagerly await to grow so that Mama can cut off the thick and delicious stems and cook them with meatballs. Our most cherished possession is the *nespra* tree, still alive and providing us with its sweet fruit. Our neighbors look down at us because we are poor and we can't afford a gardener anymore. Besides the *nespra* tree, we also have a gum tree. It was planted about three years ago and we have been using the sticky gum to starch Papa's shirts.

I can't wait for the summer so the neighbor's sweet peas can grow and climb over the cement wall, falling on our side of the yard. Then I can sit next to the wall and read my books while breathing in the summer smell of sweet peas. I also love climbing the *nespra* tree, which is my personal island. From the very top I can see the neighbors' gardens, their chicken coops, their pet dogs and cats, and further in the distance I can see other trees and houses and mountains and valleys far away in the distance. While I sit in the middle of the desert, in my oasis surrounded by *nespras* and its lush green leaves, I dream of flying away to faraway lands and travel like Gulliver and Marco Polo.

I have a serious problem in math class where we all sit in long benches next to each other because the class is so overcrowded. The girl that sits next to me keeps trying to slip her hand under my skirt. It's my fault because if I were sitting up front she wouldn't dare do that, but if I sit up front the teacher will ask me math questions, so I sit in the last row hoping not to be seen. I hate school. I hate math. I don't know who to talk to about this girl in school. When I move away from her she moves in my direction. I know that if I say something to Mama I will be in trouble for not sitting in the front row. The schoolteacher is not nice either as she was making fun of Mariana, a girl who used to be pretty before her parents punished her for misbehaving. They punished her by cutting all her long curly red hair very, very short. Now the teacher calls her unsightly and she is no longer her favorite student. I feel sorry for Mariana.

When I tried to go back into class after lunch today there was a big commotion about the tall, heavy, wood bookcase in the hallway that had fallen on top of a student. Some of the girls said another girl had gotten killed. I also heard she was taken to the hospital half alive. Nobody knows for sure and nobody knows who it was; I wonder if it was the girl that used to sit next to me. I hope she didn't die, but I do wish for her to be gone forever.

We celebrated four birthdays over the weekend. Papa is not only selling magazines but he also sells butter door to door. He must be doing very well or they borrowed the money from Aunt Heydee to buy movie tickets for the whole family. Papa's birthday was April 30, mine was May 7, Aunt Heydee is May 9 and José's will be at the end of this month. We all went to the movie theatre to see the Disney movie *Snow White*. I loved it! It was very good, but the best part was being with our parents, my brothers, and Aunt Heydee next to me. What a wonderful day it was, and to top it off at the movie theatre Papa bought the Disney book of stamps for my brothers and I and we can now spend days sticking the stamps of the movie characters in the Disney book.

Summer of 1952

Max-Leão and I heard some very alarming news while sitting on the park bench very close to where Encarnação lives. Yes, we were eavesdropping. We both wanted to know what old people talk about. Or maybe I just wanted to know it myself because I gave the idea to Max-Leão.

"Let's sit next to those two old ladies and see what they talk about."

One old lady said to the other, "It's just appalling that birthdays have to be celebrated. They should do away with birthdays. We are as young as we feel."

And the other one said, "Oh my dear, but that is exactly what's going to happen. Birthdays are just going to be a thing of the past within a few more years; no one will celebrate their birthday. After all, it's just a number."

When I got home I told the story to Mama and asked her opinion, and she said, "Don't worry, when you get to be that old you get senile and don't know what you are saying." Obviously those two ladies were very old. What a relief!

There's an old woman that lives in the building next to our house. I watch her a lot as she sits for hours on one of the benches in her backyard. She is dressed all in black from head to toe. She stares into space and talks to invisible people. Mama says that the old lady is talking to herself, because that's what happens when you get to be so old, you lose your mind. But I wonder if she is seeing something that we are not able to see.

Autumn of 1952

When I got to school today there was a line of kids having vaccines given by some doctors in white jackets. These doctors looked like the ones that took out my tonsils in the hospital a few years back. I hid behind a door and saw some kids crying as they were getting shots in their arms. I sneaked out of school and when I got home the only place I could think to hide away was under the kitchen sink. I closed the wooden doors behind me and stayed curled up until about lunchtime when I heard Mama and Aunt Heydee calling my name. The more they yelled the more I was scared and I tried to stay very still hoping for a miracle. It was going to be painful once they found me. I figured that Mama was going to beat me over the head and then later in the day I would get the same dosage from Papa. I decided that if necessary I would spend the rest of my life under the kitchen sink.

Then I heard Mama saying, "We know that you ran away from school because of the shots. I don't blame you! It's ok to come out from wherever you are hiding. I promise you don't have to have the vaccine if you don't really want it."

I came out, and after a few yells they were all laughing about my fear of needles and I didn't get hit. I was surprised that they were actually relieved and happy to see me.

Uncle Augusto made a special trip to Grandma's house just to give me the much-hated vaccine shot. It's either that or I cannot go back to school. At Mama's request, he gave me the shot on my bottom instead of my arm.

"It's bad enough that she was born with an ugly beauty mark on her abdomen," Mama said to her brother, who was insisting that the shot is normally done on the arm. She wasn't going to give up that easy, and made the argument that she was afraid that the shot might leave a scar on my arm, and men only marry women with perfect skin.

He told her he had never heard anything so dumb in his life, but had no time to quarrel with her since he was already running late.

Celeste, our part-time maid came to pick me up from school today. She told me that Mama and Papa wanted me home immediately. Lisbon was burning to the ground due to a huge fire in one of the arsenals. My brothers were already home from school. The neighbors and all of us climbed up to the very top of the black metal stairs behind our house to see the spectacular fire that was causing all kinds of fireworks. We all took turns using Papa's binoculars to see if the church next to the arsenal was in danger of getting burned. It was a beautiful sight of fiery red and yellow flames in the distance and church bells ringing, alerting everyone to get away from the fire. This is the way Rome most likely burned to the ground when the Emperor needed inspiration to play his lyre. We all took turns at using Papa's binoculars so that we could enjoy the colors of the flames up closer. Lisbon didn't burn, nobody got burned, and the church only got lots of smoke inside, so everyone agreed it was a true miracle by the grace of Saint Mary, Jesus' mother.

Last week the teacher made a hat from the daily newspaper *Diário das Noticias* and after shaping it with donkey ears she put it on my head and forced me to sit on the classroom veranda facing the street so that the people passing by could laugh at me. I thought I was going to die of shame, being seen as a donkey. It was while seated at the veranda that I developed a crying technique. I let the tears build in my eyes until they were covered with tears and I couldn't see anything.

Max-Leão has it a lot rougher than me. I learned multiplication last year, but he is having problems remembering the 7's and 8's table, and Mama is teaching him. The way she teaches is by making him repeat the multiplication tables while she sits on top of him and hits him over the head with her hands. I am surprised that he doesn't faint. I consider myself very lucky. I'd rather use a donkey hat and have people laughing at me than get beat to a pulp.

My friend, Maria Leonor, has a brain tumor. She needs brain surgery or she will die. Mama always tells me that I am a weakling and that I have weak lungs, but what Maria Leonor has sounds a lot worse. They say she might not survive the surgery, which means that she might die. Dying means you can't breathe anymore and you can't see or feel anything around you. You stop existing. You turn into dust and people walk on top of it not even realizing that they are stepping on someone's dust. I don't want to die, and I hope and pray that Maria Leonor will live. I am scared of death.

Mama likes to tell us the joke about dirt and death: Once upon a time there was a woman that didn't like cleaning her house and refused to dust. It got to a point that the dust became really thick. When a friend of hers came over to her house and realized that Maria wasn't home, she left a message on the dusty table; "Dear Maria, how many people have died in your house? There's dust everywhere!"

I used to think that was funny, but not anymore. It is a stupid story.

Aunt Morena, my mother's other sister, just came back from the island of Funchal to live in Portugal. She left her overweight, abusive husband who liked to drink beer and fool around with other women. According to Morena, her husband remarked upon seeing his newborn baby girl, "Too bad she is my daughter, she sure is going to be a beautiful girl."

Aunt Morena is waiting to be legally divorced from her monster husband who is also a catholic, and that explains why he is not a good husband as he is not a Jew. She now lives in Grandmother Rica's house with her fifteen year-old beautiful daughter, Esther, and her seventeen year old, ugly, tall, skinny, pimple-face son, Leão.

I don't like Leão. He asked me to sit on his lap and he slipped his hand up my skirt and tried to touch me between my legs. I immediately got up and I have been successful at staying away from him. I can't tell Mama. I'm afraid to get into trouble; I know that I would be blamed for it somehow. When he comes near me I spit at him, and I know that he knows why.

Winter of 1953

I just can't believe this is happening. Mama made cousin Leão my private math teacher at home. And because of him I got into serious trouble at school on Monday. Over the weekend Leão came over to our house and Max-Leão and I showed him our new blackboard hanging on the wall of our bedroom. We have white and colored chalk! We use the blackboard to write math problems, and Portuguese and French grammar, and if we make a mistake we just wipe it off with a soft flat brush, except the dust makes us cough a little when we breathe it in. José's asthma really gets messed up when he is in the room with us. The three of us like collecting as much powder as possible on the bottom shelf of the board and play with it. It's fun to make the dust fly and see it hit by the sunlight coming through the windowsills.

Cousin Leão was very impressed with our huge black board, but instead of teaching us math, he showed us instead how to draw a naked woman. All it took was six lines and a bunch of dots in the right place for the pubic hair. It was truly amazing. I can't even draw a jar in school; it always comes out crooked on one side. This was too great of an art skill not to show it off. So, on Monday when I was between classes, I gathered a few of my classmates and, trying to impress them, I drew six lines and a few dots with my black ink pen and there it was, a naked woman's body. Someone must have run out of class and snitched on me to the principal, because before I knew it I was standing in front of the class with a teacher yelling at me for producing an obscene drawing to a bunch of innocent fellow classmates. Mama was called in and I was suspended from school for a week.

That was a very good thing to happen, because when Mama found out that I had gotten the *art* lesson from cousin Leão she stopped his private tutoring with me. I couldn't tell her that Leão always found a way of putting his hand palm up on the seat just before I sat to study math with him, and it was very annoying and hard for me to concentrate on math problems when I was trying to crush his hand with my weight. He is a lousy teacher, and I hate him.

We no longer have a piano at home, but I get to hear Mama play the piano at Grandma Rica's house, and it is wonderful because children are allowed to be in the room and I can sit and hear my Aunt Heydee sing opera like Madame Butterfly and other very high-pitched singers. She makes some of the older women in the room cry because they feel sad when she sings about love and losing the one you love. I like being with everybody, but I don't care for opera with its high-pitched dramatic sound.

I love when Mama plays popular songs very fast and loud at the piano, and everybody sings along. That is a lot of fun. I get to sit on Grandma Rica's lap and I get kisses and hugs. Grandma Rica lost her husband Leão, my grandpa, many years ago, even before Mama got married. Grandpa was born in the south of Portugal. One night he had a dream about a girl that lived across the water and he would be marrying someday. So, he took the boat across the Gibraltar waters and went to Tangier to look for the girl of his dreams. While in Tangier, he was invited to a party, which happened to be at my future grandmother's parent's house. As it was customary in the old times, young girls looking to be married would come into the living room and dance or sing for their parent's guests. Rica and her sisters came into the room one at a time to meet Leão, my future grandpa. When he saw my Grandma, he immediately fell in love with her. She must have felt the same way, because they were soon married and went to Brazil to raise their family. After their first child died, they successfully had five girls, Heydee, Simy (my Mama), Nelly, Morena, Ligia, and two boys, Augusto and Abraham. They all lived in a very small village called Ticaticuaria, by the Amazon River, a long, long ride by horse-pulled carriage from the city of Manaus.

Grandpa Leão had a grocery store and a rubber plantation. He was very successful. Grandpa Leão was very kind and very smart. His name Leão, or Lion, fit him perfectly because he was very strong. When a carriage pulled by a horse fell over a man crossing the street on a rainy evening, he saved the man's life by lifting the heavy carriage with his bare hands. When a giant snake attacked a mother giving milk to her baby, he ran into the cottage after hearing her screams and pulled the snake off her and the child. He broke the snake's neck with his bare hands.

Mama remembers everything that happened in those old days when they lived in the jungles of Brazil. One of the grossest stories I heard was that once in awhile the kids were constipated and he had to slip one of his fingers into their anus and carefully pull the poop out. Kind of like unclogging the sink when it's stuck with junk.

Living by the Amazon River in those days, one had to be very careful not to fall into the hands of the Indians that shrunk heads as a prize, or cross the river when the piranha fish were swimming close by. Children are like candy to a hungry piranha. A horse and even a cow are a lot bigger than

91

a child but still they have no chance for survival if they happen to be crossing the piranha-infested river.

An interesting story happened one day when Grandma Rica was taking care of their grocery store. She cut her finger while peeling potatoes with a very sharp knife. She was alone and, not knowing what to do to stop the bleeding, she stuck her bleeding hand into the nearest open white wine barrel. It was one of those instant reactions that a person does without even thinking about it. Just then, someone came in and noticed the pink wine. "Mrs. Ezaguy, you got pink liquor now. That is incredible, please give me two full bottles of it."

She was too embarrassed to tell him what had happened. That day she sold the whole barrel of wine because everyone wanted to try the pink wine. She never again put her blood into wine; it was just an accident that turned out good.

As the years went by the ships stopped coming to Ticaticuaria and when that happened, they were impoverished and had to return to Portugal. Grandpa Leão died from a stroke when Mama was still very young; how young nobody will ever know. That's Mama's secret. She doesn't want anyone to know her present age and if anyone dares to ask her such question she will remark back by saying, "A woman is ageless and should never be asked such an offensive question."

Aunt Heydee, the eldest daughter, took over the financial burden and full responsibility of helping with the household and raising her siblings. Grandma Rica taught French, Latin, and mathematics at home but her health was not the best to be counted on. Aunt Heydee taught French and gave piano lessons privately at people's homes, and with that money she helped her family with the apartment's rent and monthly bills.

Mama has names for all our neighbors in our building; they go by what they do. The woman above us is called "drip woman" because Mama can hear the water running when she uses the bidet several times during the night. This annoys

Mama because it wakes her up. The "drip woman" real name is Rosa.

The neighbor Sofia above Rosa, on the third floor, is the "woman in black" and her two daughters are the girls of the woman in black. Sofia is a widow and black is the only color she wears since her husband died twenty years ago.

The neighbor below us is the "bad girl" and she is called that because she doesn't work and her lover who is married and with children, pays for all her living expenses. Her name is Elena.

Next to us is the "next-door woman," because she is next door. Above her are the "foreign woman" and her foreign family. We rarely see or know who lives there, they are always out traveling. On the floor directly above them nobody knows who lives there. "The renters" are the ones below our next-door neighbor. There's always someone new moving in, and as soon as we learn their name, they move out.

I have gotten into trouble again. I'm going to lose my best friend Encarnação. What am I going to do? But I didn't lie. I was spending the afternoon at Encarnação's home with her niece Laura. We were both sitting at Encarnação's tea table with the hot coal below our feet and Laura was reading a book while I was studying my grammar. Then a man came in, it was Laura's boyfriend because he called her honey, and they kissed on the lips. While they were seated on the couch, he kept trying to put his hands into her blouse but I made believe that I wasn't seeing anything. He said they were going to the kitchen to make me tea. They left the room and later they brought me tea and cookies.

While I was seated at the table, they both sat on the floor and he tried to put his hands under her skirt. She kept asking him to stop and pushing his hands away, looking at me embarrassed.

Finally I said, "Stop that, don't you see that she doesn't want you to touch her that way."

He got angry and told me to shut up and keep studying. She asked him to leave and he did.

When I got home I told Mama what happened, and she must have told Encarnação and the result was both of them said that I had exaggerated what I had seen and as such I was damaging her niece Laura's reputation and conduct. I am so embarrassed over this; I didn't mean to hurt anyone. I just thought that if Mama spoke to Encarnação then she could protect Laura from that man. I have to learn not to react to other people's problems, and most of all, not to tell Mama anything.

For a couple of months, a ghost has been knocking at Grandmother Rica's door. That is the only explanation according to neighbors, friends, and family, because every time they open the door there's nobody there. This is very, very, very scary. The knock can happen in the middle of the night or anytime during the day. A policeman was hired to stand behind the closed door and wait for the knock, and the neighbors were on the lookout, but no luck. It all started after Christmas. It looks like it is a ghost because while the policeman was there the knocks stopped, then started again, when he left. After months of sleepless nights, Grandma Rica and everybody in the house are becoming nervous wrecks.

What a relief! The ghost was the neighbor downstairs! They were trying to scare Grandma to move out so that their daughter who is getting married in April could move into the apartment above them. Aunt Heydee was the one that discovered the plot. Without telling anyone she drilled a hole from inside the closet wall facing the steps to Grandma's front door and with a flashlight in hand she spent a few nights awake looking through the hole to the outside. Sure enough she saw the husband's neighbor running up the stairs. After knocking at the door he would run up to the next flight of steps so that he would not get caught, but Aunt Heydee saw it all and called the police. His wife cried for mercy and Grandma felt sorry for the "ghost's wife," so he was told to stop and was not arrested. From all the embarrassment, there's talk that the "ghost family" will be moving out soon.

I like reading the comic books at Sofia's house, our neighbor on the third floor. I can only read them when I am visiting her. She won't allow me to take them with me to read at home. But that's okay. I have learned to enjoy the smell of her apartment; furniture wax mixed with garlic, vinegar, and cleaning fluid. She doesn't talk too much; she looks sad in her black dress, black apron, black socks and black shoes. She stays busy cleaning the house and she leaves me alone to read the comics in her sunroom.

My favorite comic book is about the old prairie man that lived in the desert of Arizona in North America. He was very old, about a hundred and five years old, so he no longer could kill buffaloes. One day he got sick from old age and everyone was outside his tent waiting to see if he was going to live or die, but of course everyone knew that he was going to die very soon, because nobody lives past a hundred and five. Then as everyone came into his tent and surrounded his bed looking anxiously at him, he sat up and said, "Present!" And he took a deep breath and, falling peacefully on his back, he was dead. He had gone to God without suffering. I hope I drop dead too, when I have to die.

Grandmother Rica has new neighbors. The other neighbors are in an uproar, complaining because their neighborhood is becoming low-class and they can't do anything about it. The apartment where the "ghost" family used to live has been rented out to very beautiful older girls, barely covered with colorful silk robes, and busy opening their front door to strange men. When that happens, while I am going up the steps to visit Grandma, I am to turn my head the other way, and I'm not allowed to look in that direction, but I peek to the left side and they always say hello to me and smile. I heard that these girls play with men's penises to give them pleasure and they get paid very well for it. A lot of the men visiting them are married men and they go there because their wives are not perverted and refuse to give their husbands perverted sex and this is the only way they can get it, when they pay for it. According to Mama, her sisters, and her girlfriends, only single men should be allowed to visit these girls and if anything the whole whorehouse should be in another part of town and not right under Grandma's house.

I was playing yesterday on the lower steps of Grandma Rica's house with my two younger cousins Sonia and Elsinha when a fat ugly old man with moles on his face walked into the hallway and as he walked up the steps he pinched Sonia's buttocks very hard. She was crying after that and the man just laughed as he knocked at the "girls" door and a pretty girl in a pink silk robe let him in. We all ran upstairs to Grandma who was very upset over what happened, but nothing could be done about it.

I like being helpful, but when I try to be nice I get into trouble. I am clumsy. I am defective and I have known that for a long time. Something is wrong with me. I don't know exactly what, yet. I can tell that I am different from everybody else; I can also tell everyone else is a lot smarter than me.

I was visiting Sofia, as I always do when I have nothing else to do. I like sitting in her guestroom reading the comic books she has kept through the years from when her children were younger. She doesn't throw anything away. I also like to follow her around the rooms as she dusts and shines her silver platters and silverware. Her apartment is very clean and organized. Her two daughters are all grown up and don't visit her as often as she would like them to. Her husband died a long time ago. She lives alone and she doesn't mind when I come over. I have never seen her bake any cakes or sweets. Her kitchen never smells of vanilla or toasted almonds or chocolate melting, like at Encarnação's kitchen. Sofia doesn't like sunshine and her wooden shutters are always closed. When she is in the kitchen she is always busy grinding meat in the metal grinder or soaking rabbits in vinegar or boiling snails with garlic and olive oil. Sofia always puts a few snails in a plate for me to eat. I love snails. I use one of her safety pins to pull the little creatures out, very tasty indeed. She never offers me other food, just snails; thank God because I would not eat rabbit, that's for sure. I have never seen a skinned cat, but I bet you couldn't tell the difference if they were skinned side by side. So, there I was watching her cutting some meat and putting it through the meat grinder when suddenly she couldn't turn the handle, the wheel inside the grinder was stuck with all the meat and gristle inside of it and would not roll over. She was cursing the grinder and life because she had to pull the whole grinding machine apart, so I decided to give her some of my expert advice. I asked her why she did not use a knife to pull the meat out, like my mother does. Just stick it inside like this — and I showed her how and — I twisted the knife inside the roller blades — and broke the knife inside the grinder. She yelled at me and told me never to come back to her house again.

A whole week has gone by, and Sofia sent me a message downstairs that I should come and visit her. She had made me something very special. I was relieved to find out that she was still my friend. She had prepared my favorite dish, a batch of snails. But she had bought giant snails with long antennas and I simply could not put one in my mouth. I would have to be a cannibal to eat something that big. She kept saying, "C'mon, try it. I got the big ones this time, just for you. Don't you like them?"

It was gross and plain disgusting; how can anyone eat those creatures when they are huge and have long antennas? I didn't want to hurt Sofia's feelings, so I made believe that I was eating them, by putting them in my mouth, but carefully stuffing them to the sides of my mouth. When she left the room I ran out the back door and spat out a mouth full of snails into the downstairs neighbor's yard.

Mama got a call from Encarnação. Maria Leonor's surgery to remove the brain tumor was a success and she is back from the hospital, alive — but blind. I was invited to stop by and say hello to Maria Leonor. Luisa, our part-time maid, went with me.

As we entered Encarnação's home we both backed away when we saw Maria Leonor. What had happened to my once beautiful play friend? Her long blonde hair had been shaved off and there was a big nasty scar in her skull. She was standing there looking into space, emaciated and surrounded by darkness. Luisa grabbed my arm as she backed away, horrified. I didn't recognize Maria Leonor except for her eyes that were still blue, and her smile still soft and without anger as she said, "Is that you Verónica?"

My stomach twisted inside out and I though that I was going to throw up. Then I picked up my courage and went up to her and hugged her even though I was scared that what she had was contagious. She was horrible to look at as if she was dead. I didn't cry until I left their house. I am better off being plain, even dumb. I don't care anymore if I am really nothing special to look at, but I can see. My hair is dark brown and my eyes are green, thank you God for that. I feel fine the way I am, any color; doesn't matter and I promise that I will never be jealous of anyone, never again.

Later today Mama told me that Encarnação had called to tell her that she was very impressed with me because I had hugged Maria Leonor, and the maid had backed away. That meant that I had a good heart. I didn't tell Mama that I don't have a good heart, and I didn't hug Maria Leonor because I am good. I did it because I thought that if it were me it would be nice to have a hug from a friend. I was really afraid to catch her blindness but I didn't want her to know how horrible she looked. I didn't want to hurt her feelings. If I didn't hug her, she would also know that she looked totally disgusting and I couldn't do that. I am sad and ashamed to feel this way about my best and only friend. I don't feel good about my feelings this morning. I am selfish.

Maria Leonor.

I told Mama what happened the other day when I visited Sofia. Now I am not allowed to visit Sofia anymore. I shouldn't have told Mama about it but my feelings were hurt. What happened is that Sofia was having a friend over for tea and I was seated on the floor reading some magazines when Sofia said to her friend, "Do you smell something — like a smelly fart?"

"Now that you mention it - yeah, I guess so."

"Verónica, come here," and as I approached Sofia she said, "Are you being a disgusting little girl by passing gas in our presence?" And before I could even reply that it wasn't me, she grabbed me and pulled my skirt up and took a sniff at my underwear saying, "Yep it's you alright, get out of here and go home."

I left, crying of course, because I knew I didn't smell bad and I knew I had no gas either. It had to be her or her friend, but it wasn't me. I had to tell Mama about it because I don't like to be called a liar unless it's true.

I brought home three of my girl friends from school to play with me. I could only play with them in our backyard. Mama is ashamed of our house, empty of furniture with decaying walls and closets. One of the girls asked me if she could use our bathroom. I went running in and asked Mama if Joana could use our bathroom.

Mama's response was, "Tell her to go home and use her own bathroom, this is not a public bathroom."

I was so embarrassed that Joana was not allowed to come in to use our bathroom. She said she would never make it all the way home and she made poop in one of the corners of our yard while we all looked the other way. Later that day Mama made me go in the yard and remove the poop with some newspapers. I don't like Mama anymore; she is mean.

Spring of 1953

Last Sunday, Luisa took me to visit her family. They live in Alfama, the poorest borough of Lisbon. The house was very old and small but very clean and smelled of green vegetable soup, my favorite. With each spoonful I like to take my time and suck the mashed potatoes between my teeth and that way I am able to maintain the finely chopped collard greens in between my lips and front teeth. I do that because I like the taste and chewing the collard greens at the end.

Then Julio, her spastic nephew who is six years old, so they said, came in the room and decided to look under my skirt. He didn't even tell me. He just lifted my skirt and stuck his head under it so I pulled him out, made a fist, and knocked him out.

When I got home I heard nothing but abuse because I took advantage of a little boy. I should have been more understanding. Give me a break! Any boy, small or big, if he pulls my skirt up to look up at my private parts is going to be knocked out cold.

Summer of 1953

I get to spend a lot of Sundays with Grandma Rica. She helps me with math and French, my two worst subjects in school. I don't like either. They are both boring. Spending the day with Grandma is like being in school, no time to play or simply have fun. I love hugging her and playing with her wrinkled hands, which I wish I had, but I don't want to spend my free time learning school stuff. She put me in her bedroom and closed the door and told me that I could not play with my brothers until I studied more. My goodness, it's summer time and I need some time off from using my brain. I am on vacation and this means I should be playing and having fun. I cried because I was angry, frustrated and jealous that Max-Leão and José were playing in her kitchen. Studying French is like learning math, a brain torture. I

101

wished that Grandma Rica would die, and then I could be free to go out and play.

I like sunshine but I don't get along with too much heat, as I found out when I spent the day yesterday with Aunt Heydee at Estoril, her favorite beach. As always, Aunt Heydee knows how to find a free lounge chair available to sit on at the esplanade under one of their large umbrellas by the water, where everyone who has money sits and sips ultra-expensive cold drinks. I didn't play in the water or take a walk on the rocky cliffs. I just sat there next to her all afternoon. It's always fun watching the people go by and listening to Aunt Heydee's interesting conversations with whoever sits next to her. It was a hot, slightly hazy, lazy day and the sun never really came out from behind the clouds.

This morning I got up and went to the bathroom next to my bedroom — when I come home, my room can be anywhere in the house, Mama is always changing the furniture from one room to another. I sat on the toilet and passed out. I came back to the world with my face burning from being slapped and I was lying in bed shivering.

Uncle Augusto told Mama that I had a heat stroke from being at the beach yesterday. From now on I have to use a hat in the sun and if it's too hot I am to stay inside the coolest place around. I am a weakling, a good-for-nothing. I would never make it if I had to cross the desert or got shipwrecked and found myself on a deserted island without the shade of palm trees. The city is too hot in the summertime. Our only relief is to go to the beach at least once a week and cool off in the ocean. It's healthy to be near the ocean and breathe in the salty air. Everybody says the salty ocean water kills all illnesses. We can only afford the train ticket to the smelly beach of Oeiras, not too far from Lisbon. As soon as you exit the train you can't miss the strong whiff of raw sewage. The small village of Oeiras must be dumping their sewage directly into the ocean and onto their beach. The Oeiras population must be very poor because nobody cares to fix the problem. My brothers and I like to play in the sand, building sand castles, but we are not allowed in the water because it's too polluted, which makes no difference since we can't swim anyway. Our only fun is catching the small purple ocean creatures that wash ashore and squeezing their purple ink out. We have contests to see who squeezes the most ink out of each one.

Aunt Heydee has taken me a few times to Cascais and Estoril; these are the only two beaches she will visit because she likes to mingle with the rich and more intellectual people. There are no foul smells at those beaches. The air smells of salt, seaweed, tobacco, tanning lotions, and perfumes the rich foreigners bring in from their countries.

My favorite park used to be the Cesário Verde, by Encarnação's house, but it has turned into a park for adults only. I used to like it a lot because it was small, and not too far from home so I was allowed to go there and play by myself or with my two brothers. I especially liked to roll on the grass from the top of the center mound and down the little hill until I hit the ground below. Then one day the new gardener removed the smooth grassy hill and covered it with spiky plants, flowers and bushes. None of us kids can use the hill to roll down. Our playground has been destroyed. A bunch of wooden benches have been added for people that need to sit. Nothing lasts forever.

I spend many afternoons at the Park Estefania, a few blocks from our house. I sit there for hours reading the books they have in their outside library and for the most part nobody bothers me. Then one afternoon, I noticed some girls and boys my age improvising on stories, like Cinderella and Little Red Riding Hood. One of them came up to me and asked me if I would play with them, I said yes. But soon I found that we needed a director and since I was the only one volunteering I did it gladly. We have been gathering every Wednesday and Friday after lunch to perform for ourselves. It has been my passion this summer. Following the pattern of the story, and with imagination as our friend, we make fantasies become a reality.

Autumn of 1953

When Grandmother Rica was young she belonged to the Masons. Mama told me that her mother belonged to this group of secret people that helped others less fortunate and if it weren't for her they would have died. Grandmother Rica had been a spy for France during World War I. She was one of the very rare women that were accepted as a member of this secret society because of her education. Besides being proficient in many languages like Hebrew, Arabic, Spanish, Portuguese, English, and French, she was a wizard at math. She used to travel with her father as his secretary and bookkeeper, and it was while she was in France that she was inducted into the Masons and become an active member. When she got married with Grandpa Leão she burned all the secret papers and buried what was left in her backyard. She could not divulge the names of the people she had worked with.

Aunt Heydee became the breadwinner at a young age. After her father's death and her mother being sick, Aunt Heydee felt that as the eldest it was her obligation to see to it that her family was cared for. With a family to care for, she could only pay for one of her two brothers' education. She had to choose between Abraham and Augusto. Because Augusto was smarter than Abraham, she took Augusto under her wing and paid for his tuition through medical school while my mother and her sister Ligia continued their studies at the Conservatory of Music.

Aunt Heydee's nickname is Napoleão, because if she had been born a man she would have conquered the world. She has never been married and she will not settle for anything less than what she deserves, therefore no one is perfect enough for her. He has to be religious, rich, handsome, young, intelligent, sensitive, yet strong and — most of all — has to like opera. She is not only the breadwinner of the house, but she is the oldest of all the brothers and sisters, and she takes this position very seriously. Everybody respects her because she knows everything. On the wedding night Aunt

Ligia and her husband were having problems consummating their marriage because she was a virgin, whatever that means, so they called Aunt Heydee that night on the phone and asked her for advise. She told Ligia and her new husband to use a pillow under her bottom and to relax while having sex on the hard floor instead of the soft bed. After that Ligia got pregnant. I learn a lot from sitting next to adults and hearing their conversations.

Grandmother Rica fell down the other day. I heard that she is bleeding inside and might die. She is very old and nothing can be done about it they say. I went to see her; she was lying down on her right side facing the wall. I kissed her face and she didn't even move. I am scared. I do not want her to die. Please God, I didn't mean for her to die, I just wanted to have time off to play. I say stupid things all the time because I was born stupid. I hate myself.

Grandmother Rica died. I cried as hard as I could today. The more my eyes were burning from the tears the better I felt. I was hoping that I could go blind like Maria Leonor. Never again will I see my Grandmother's smile and kind look, as she would give me bread with bananas or homemade orange-peel jam. No longer can I play with her wrinkled hands. She will never hold me close again. I want to die too.

Mama asked Papa to take me in his *lambretta*, a small motorcycle that he bought used and it's very cheap on gasoline. The ride will dry my tears away, she told him. Going for the ride and holding on to Papa made me feel better.

He said that from now on he would take me with him on business trips around Portugal because I am his oldest child and I liked riding the motorcycle with him. He is going to teach me how to read maps.

I heard Mama and Aunt Heydee talking about their brother, Uncle Augusto. He gave Grandmother Rica a special injection so that she could die in peace. She was in too much pain and nothing could be done to save her. He is a very kind doctor, and he also loved his mother a lot and couldn't bear to see her suffer when nothing could be done medically to save her. I hope I get to be old like my Grandmother someday, but I don't want to suffer for many days before I die either. Mama likes to tell everybody how she was blessed because she held her mother in her arms as Grandmother Rica took her last breath.

Winter of 1954

Sometimes after school is over, some of my school friends take me along to the church across the street. The church is a tall simple white building, with lots of white marble steps leading to a dark wooden double-door. The inside is dark and it takes a while to get your eyes used to the only available light coming from the smelly candles and narrow dusty rays of sunlight squeezing through the only two small stained-glass windows, as if daring to take no for an answer. It is always dark and smelly inside this church and the stone walls inside are covered with saints made of wood and marble, dressed in gold and adorned with precious stones.

It is a community church and it doesn't have the splendor of the big churches made for large amounts of people like the one Encarnação took me to during last Easter's festivities when I got to kiss Jesus' feet. That church was so big that we both stayed in line all morning before we finally made it to the altar. Even though Jesus was made of wood, Mama had a fit when she found out. Mama blamed me for going to church with Encarnação. I should have refused to go. I was grounded for one month and I was not allowed to visit Encarnação. This is not fair, Encarnação just wanted me to see her God and she was sharing him with me. I will always love Encarnação.

Every year, probably to welcome spring, about a dozen poor brides are married at the community church, all at the same time. Their expenses, honeymoon trip, dresses, and the rest are all paid for by business people as a form of advertisement that not only promotes their business as being run by good and kind people but also helps to keep these girls in line for marriage and with good morals, which is what all Catholic girls are encouraged to do before they get old and become spinsters like my Aunt Heydee.

My friends at school are Catholic and they are going to Heaven and they want me to go to Heaven too when I die. They have told me over and over again that if I repent, and become a Catholic instead of being Jewish, Jesus would forgive me for having killed him. I have told them time and time again that I had nothing to do with it.

My two best friends Maria José and Josefina say that if I go to church with them after school I have a better chance of going to Heaven. I want them to be my friends, so I go to church with them at least twice a week. I don't want to offend them, but this church is very depressing with lots of dead people in stone coffins above ground and under the church floor. You have to step over them in order to walk inside the church, very creepy indeed.

The people who lived a long time ago are now saints made of stone. Sinners now pray for forgiveness on their knees, praying to these statues and asking for miracles. There are also lots of dark paintings with scenes of Jesus, a man that was crucified on the cross, and his mother, and other saints suffering with him and fat little angels all around.

The old and pale priest dressed in black walks inside the church rolling a necklace of beads between his fingers. He never smiles and speaks a foreign language called Latin. I don't know what he says when he does his sermon while we sit on the hard benches. The smell of candles and incense gives me a headache just like when my friend Encarnação fixes my hair back into a bunion on top of my head. Confession is very important, my girl friends told me; you must confess every week to the priest behind the curtain.

I asked them, "What if you don't have anything to confess?"

They told me they have to make it up otherwise they will be going to Hell. I don't want to be a Catholic if I have to lie for God to love me.

When Mama has company she always tries to impress her guests. My brothers and I come into the living room, and then she asks the big question, "Tell everyone, where babies come from?"

All three of us say it in a chorus effect, "From big huge sunflowers!"

Mama and her guests giggle and go, "Ah, they sure are innocent!"

I have known that this is not true for quite some time. I am a good listener at Mama's gatherings with her sisters and I collect a lot of information about life in general, including a lot of our family history. But since it makes Mama happy, I don't have the courage to tell her that I feel like a retard every time I have to act ignorant. What I don't know is how the baby got inside the belly in the first place.

I have been looking for God but I have not been able to find Him. Mama took me to the temple a few months ago but I didn't see God there either. This is the only Jewish Temple in Lisbon and it's hidden behind a large metal door. Even the neighbors next to it don't know there's a temple next to them. Mama told me the reason it is this way is because of prejudice. If it's not seen, people with other religious beliefs can't destroy it. They think only their God is good. They are called fanatics. So our temple is not like a church where everybody going by can make the cross across his or her chest. Also, our temple doesn't have saints on the walls or buried dead people inside tombs. Our temple is very simple inside except for the really nice dark mahogany chairs. The temple was built for praying only. The men pray downstairs and the women sit upstairs so there are no distractions while praying to God. It does have a medium size niche with doors, almost like an altar to God but when they open the doors to it there are no stone saints inside nailed to crosses like in

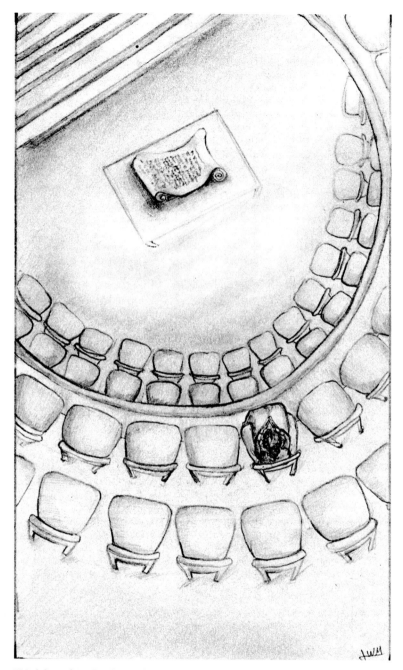

Waiting for God to Show Up.

Church. Inside are the rolled manuscripts with words from God. I believe it's the Bible, but it's written in Hebrew, so I don't know what they are saying when they read it out loud. I have been keeping my eyes and ears open at the temple and when I first saw a ray of sunshine coming through one of the small windows I was hoping that was going to be it, but I don't believe that was God.

I admire the people praying inside; they must know something I don't. God must be invisible, just like Mama and Papa have told me so many times. Being invisible has to be a good thing. I would love to be invisible, then I could go into a candy store and eat all the candy and chocolate I wish. I was at the temple last week and got bored listening to the rabbi, (he has the same type of job as the priest in the Catholic Church) and the men below us praying in Hebrew, a very strange language. I have no idea what they were saying; it sounds a lot like German. They move their bodies back and forth as if they are dancing to the sound of their voices, and they never look up to look at the women. They are very religious. I don't understand why God doesn't understand Portuguese and can only be spoken to in foreign languages like Hebrew or Latin.

I made a big mistake! I told Mama about my visits to church with my friends from school. She gave me a big lecture about us being Jews and that it is a sin for us to enter a Catholic church. We have endured a lot of suffering and prosecution through the ages and during World War II.

Our ancestors would have wasted their lives in misery and abuse for nothing if I were to become a Catholic. I am not to date a Catholic and when I get married it will be to a Jew so that my children will be Jewish, otherwise my children will also marry Catholics and our religion will be lost forever.

Mama hung a picture of my two cousins from Germany on my bedroom wall. They were very pretty girls, dressed in white organza dresses with big matching white bows properly set up on their long brown curly hair. One is seated by her piano while the other stands holding a flute. They are both smiling at the photographer; they look like angels should look. They are only a few years older than I. They were eleven and twelve years old when they were taken to a concentration camp. They were the only two daughters of my father's youngest sister, Ilse. The story goes that upon the rising of Hitler to power, her husband ran away, abandoning her and the children in Germany. She arranged to save her children first by sending them to a school in Holland, thinking they would be safe there. She didn't expect the Nazis to invade Holland and take away all the children from that school into a concentration camp. All these years, Ilse has been writing to the Russian government, to find out if their soldiers took her daughters to Russia when they attacked Germany. Until today her letters have never been answered.

Mama gave us an anatomy book, where all the parts of the body just pop out from the page. When I looked at Max-Leão who had been standing next to me as I flipped the pages, he was flat on the floor. He fainted when he saw the inside of a pregnant woman's belly with a baby inside of her.
     Mama informed us that it's called a fetus. Mama must have realized that it was time for us to learn where babies come from. I already knew that but when I asked her how the baby got inside the belly, she said I was too young to know.

Spring of 1954

Mama brought home a clay pot with red and white carnations, Grandmother Rica's favorite flowers, and she put the container under the *nespra* tree. I see Mama watering the carnations just about every day with a tin can and she cries. She really misses her mother. I miss my grandmother too.

Sofia, our upstairs neighbor on the third floor, died from a stroke. She went into a coma for about two weeks. The whole neighborhood was praying for her recovery. I wanted to go upstairs to see her. She was my snail connection, and my silent friend, except for when she falsely accused me of making farts. But I already forgave her for that; it wasn't that important anyway. Mama would not allow me to see Sofia, saying that she was dying and that was no place for children. I was very sad after Sofia died. I will never see her again.

After they took Sofia's body away, I went to visit her oldest daughter who was living in Sofia's apartment. Angela spoke of her mother with tenderness while washing her own personal underwear in the bathroom sink; they were made of silk and of different colors, not black. She told me that it was okay to have colorful underwear, as long as she wore black dresses to cover them in respect for her mother's death; besides, it was just underwear and that didn't represent how she felt in her heart.

I told Mama how beautiful Angela's colorful underwear was. Mama said it was terrible that Angela wore colorful underwear. After all, her mother had died not even a month ago. Not wearing black was disrespectful.

I don't agree. I think that colorful underwear should be optional.

We were having lunch when Mama got a codfish bone stuck inside her throat once again. We all ran out of the apartment on the way to the first aid squad when the neighbors below us and the porter and his wife, living below them, upon hearing the commotion, came out.

"What's wrong, Mrs. Wartenberg?"

Out of embarrassment Mama put her fingers down her throat and in desperation she pulled the bone out, responding as rapidly as possible, "Nothing is wrong; I was just checking, I thought I heard the doorbell ring."

And she ran back up the steps and into the apartment, saying, "I wasn't going to let them rejoice at seeing me choke to death."

The porter and his wife have made a list of offensive acts on our part, like not taking care of our yard, making too much noise when my brothers and I play, not closing the door downstairs when we come into the building, or closing the door downstairs too hard, all petty stuff. The landlord is trying to throw us out so that he can rent our apartment for more money. But the law protects us as long as we pay the rent even if it's at the last moment.

Papa would never choke on a fishbone, because he is an expert German fish eater. I have choked a couple of times on the very thin bones, but I coughed really hard until they came out. I hope Papa never chokes on a fish bone. He would be so humiliated.

I won't be going to high school very soon. I have finished the four grades needed to enter high school, but our parents cannot afford to send Max-Leão and me to school at the same time. I would have to go to a private girl's school, and they can't afford the expense. Mama doesn't want to take any chances that I might meet and marry a goim, (a Catholic). Max-Leão is not only smarter than me but he is going to be a man, therefore he will have to have an education so that he can work and take care of his family. Mama said I would be getting married to my cousin Alberto from North America; so I don't need to be educated. My husband will take care of me. Besides, if I go to public high school I will most likely fall in love with a *goim*, and if that were to happen it would be the end of our religion from my side.

Max-Leão will go to an all-boy's school, only for a couple of years, and then at fifteen years old he will be sent to England were our cousins will make sure he goes to college and become an architect, which is what seems to be his inclination. When he gets married he has to work and be able to provide for his own family. Our family in England has the finances to help him towards a good career.

"Our parents have set up our future," I told Max-Leão just before we dozed off to sleep last night. We like to talk about many wonderful things before falling asleep. Our favorite subject is fantasizing about an earthquake and we both get stuck under the entire rubble of a building for a week. Of course, we would like to be inside a candy store or a bakery when an earthquake hits Lisbon someday.

Summer of 1954

We are spending two months in Costa da Caparica, a huge beach across the river Tejo. We all got here on the back of a small pick-up truck. My brothers and I were sandwiched between the pots and pans, mattresses, some furniture, and boxes of clothing. It was a very bumpy and windy trip and a few times I thought one of us was going to be part of the asphalt road. But we need everything we brought along, because the place we are staying doesn't have anything except four walls, a door and a wood stove.

This is not a beach for sissies like, Cascais and Estoril, which are beaches for tourists and city people that don't really want to travel far. This beach is for the people of Portugal; clean, sparkly sand for hundreds of miles. I already tried to walk to the end and gave up after hours and hours of walking. Most likely it keeps going until it reaches the Algarve way down in the south of Portugal. It was from the Algarve that the great Portuguese navigators made history when they left to conquer the world. Mama found our little cement shack for absolutely peanuts to rent. The days are always the same; we get up, make the bed, get into the bathing suit, have a tall glass of coffee and milk in equal parts, and a *papo seco* (a small bread very close to French bread), and run to the beach to play, carrying the lunch bag, a bottle of water, a towel, a small tin bucket and a spatula for building our castles and "the nail," my favorite sand game.

We have our own white cloth tent that we rent for the whole time we are on vacation. Everybody has one, even the people that are here just for one day. It's used to store everything we have with us when we leave to play in the water. When the sun is too hot, we seek shade inside the tent we call *cabana*. Our *cabana* makes a great place to nap after

Going Away for the Summer.

lunch, even though it can get very hard to breathe without any fresh air inside. I usually lay down on the outside on the side of shade where a breeze somehow passes by me. All the cabanas are made with four wood poles that stick into the sand. They are covered on all sides, including the top, with a white thick cloth-like material. When you want to leave your valuables inside and go swimming, the front gets dropped and tied to the sides with rope.

Our valuables are food, towels, and water. Our lunch usually consists of fried fish and rice, or codfish cakes — which are potatoes and codfish, minced garlic, eggs and parsley, mashed together and molded into small cakes and then fried and served with fresh lemon. I don't like eating fried food because I always get nauseous afterwards. I would rather have salad or fruit, whatever is in season, but we can't afford these luxuries. We are lucky to have codfish and potatoes every day.

During the week, Papa stays in Lisbon working. He only comes over to visit us on Saturday afternoon and then leaves Sunday evening, back to the city. He has to work very hard in order to pay for our food, our stay at the beach for the summer, and all the daily things we need. I feel that Mama should be working with Papa by his side instead of staying at the beach with us. I feel she is selfish, but I am not saying anything. I admire Papa for not giving up on all of us and working so hard, but that doesn't change the fact that I am afraid of talking or being near him. He never shows me any affection and Mama never hugs me either. My brothers are her favorite children; José is the youngest and always sick so he is definitely her favorite, Max-Leão ranks second in her heart. I am not loved by anyone. But on the other hand, my parents no longer hit me as often as they used to, and for the most part they leave me alone to do whatever I like, mostly reading. I intend to read every book I can get my hands on this summer.

Last night we went to bed without dinner. One of the soap boxes kept on a shelf above the stove fell into the open soup pot and no matter how much Mama tried to scoop out the soap bubbles, it just wasn't eatable, so we all went to bed hungry. Even though there isn't enough space for all of us in this house, I don't mind sleeping in the kitchen with my two brothers. Mama feels very embarrassed to be staying in this place and hopes that no one she knows will see us living here. I am very glad to be here and I don't care where I sleep as long as we have something to eat everyday.

I believe that Mama has gained a certain kind of wisdom that has grown out of her personal experiences in life. She no longer gets upset about losing material things.

Her favorite statement for everything that goes wrong is, "Better to lose the diamond rings than your fingers."

I agree with that, but why lose anything at all?

Last night Max-Leão and I spent the evening peeling off the skin from under each other's feet. Not a good idea. We had to stay home today. We can't walk because the soles of our feet are very painful to walk on, so we read some books and then spent the rest of the day peeling the skin off our backs.

Mama believes that if she stands in front of the ocean waves when they crash for as long as she can bear them hitting her body, they will beat the fat out of her body and she will lose weight. I don't think that's going to happen unless she stops eating. She is always pointing to other women that look bigger than her, but to me she doesn't look any smaller than them. I think it has to do with her eating so many raw eggs with sugar. I don't blame her though; it is the best dessert I can think of. She beats the raw yellow of the egg with sugar, and keeps putting sugar until it changes into a paste of just the right consistency. Then she adds pieces of bread to it and mashes it down with a spoon, and eats it like a cake. I believe this is a Spanish delicacy, because every time Uncle Augusto travels to Spain, he brings me a little wood barrel filled with egg and sugar. Last time he went to Spain he brought me a silver bracelet, which was very nice of him, and I do like it a lot, but

Soap Soup.

I miss the little barrel of sugar and egg. Mama said the reason he brought me a bracelet instead is because I am a grown girl, not a baby anymore. What does a little barrel of egg with sugar have to do with me being grown up? I still like it.

We can't afford treats, but Mama found someone that was selling rennet apples by the box, and we now have enough apples for the whole month as long as we have only one each day. The apples are kept on the floor under my bed, where the stone kitchen floor keeps them fresh. I love the aroma coming from under my bed. I feel like I am sleeping on top of an apple orchard.

The days are very relaxing at the beach. Playing with my brothers, making holes in the sand and covering them with newspapers then with sand, just enough to hide the newspapers. Then we wait for a victim while we hide inside our *cabana*, laughing our heads off and hoping that someone will fall into the hole. We have not had any luck so far, and this is a bit disappointing. We make sand castles and other artistic shapes out of sand like people and boats. We dig huge holes and take turns burying each other up to our heads in the sand, just like in Arabia when the warriors would ride their horses and with a quick sweep of their swords, cut their enemies' heads off. When you are buried in the hot sunny desert of Arabia with just your head sticking out you know your luck just ran out.

We spend endless hours just trying to outdo each other with stories and games, particularly the nail game. The purpose of the nail game is to get the nail to land straight and upright into the sand after some ingenious moves with sliding it off our elbows to other creative moves like interlacing it between the fingers. After we have our lunch of fried codfish cakes and bread we have the midday nap inside our *cabana*.

We have started to relax on the water and because we are less afraid we now are able to float on our backs as long as the ocean is calm and there are no waves to run over us. We even ride the small waves on our tummies, but neither of us is swimming far into the ocean like other people do. Then Mama had the great idea of paying a beach boy to take my brothers and me into the ocean. Why? Because it's good for us! The nasty bastard took José, who was smaller, under one of his arms, and Max-Leão and I followed him innocently, having no idea what was about to happen. He was supposed to be teaching us to swim. When he got to an area where the water was to his waist, he threw José into the water and pushed him under. Max-Leão took off as fast as a bullet and I tried to do the same, but the beach boy grabbed me by the hair and pushed me under also. Gasping for air, I swallowed lots of water and thought I was going to drown. Somehow I slipped out off his hands and between swimming and running, and by a miracle of God, I got to the shore where I cried and cried as I lay on the sand. I was screaming at the top of my lungs, cursing him, Mama, and the whole world of stupid nasty people around me.

I no longer make holes in the sand and wait for people to fall into one of them. Whatever I do to someone, it will sooner or later happen to me. I fell into a hole in the sand. Some stupid kids were playing the same prank as my brothers and I. My ankle got twisted as I fell into it, and they laughed as if it was a big joke. No, it's not a joke I didn't laugh. It's so embarrassing to fall in front of strangers. I told my brothers about it and they thought it was funny. I am staying away from them when they are digging. I will not be part of it anymore. Besides, it is absolutely childish.

It's almost time to go back to Lisbon; we have to be back to the city by the end of this month. Mama spends a lot of time in the sun and we don't see each other unless it's lunchtime or dinner.

I was very sick a few days ago with fever and a stomachache. I was lying down in bed and Mama came to me and put her hand on my head, saying, "Verónica, you are going to be fine."

I started to cry with happiness. Her hand on my head was like being in Heaven, but I didn't say anything. I just closed my eyes; I didn't want her to think that I was a weakling begging for her love. The pain was gone and I fell asleep.

Autumn of 1954

According to Mama, I have so far had every illness known to children. Nope, it doesn't matter if I got vaccinated or not, and right now everybody at home has the mumps. I gave it to them. Even Mama and Papa are sick with it. We all have big chins, except Max-Leão. He says he refuses to catch it and that's it. Mama is worried about him, because, according to her brother Augusto, it's better to have the mumps while you are young; in particular men, because they can become sterile if they catch this disease while adults. This means that Papa is now sterile too, which makes no sense since men don't have babies anyway. But whatever that means, he no longer can be a father again. Mama went on a mission to make Max-Leão catch the mumps. She kisses him in the mouth every day and that is what I call disgusting. She even had him sleep with her so that she would breathe on him all night long, but he kept saying, "No I won't catch it!"

I admire my brother. When he puts his mind to it, he really sticks with it. I wish I were like him. He is so smart.

Uncle Augusto has diagnosed me with juvenile rheumatoid arthritis. That's why I get horrible pain in my legs. I was born this way. Sometimes it hurts very sharp like knives sticking into my bones. Uncle Augusto is always giving me medicine but it doesn't help at all. Mama makes me sit in the backyard with my legs in the sun, she says the heat is good for it, but that doesn't help either. The only thing that helps just a little is rubbing my legs, but they have to be rubbed really hard so that it hurts more than the bone pain. I cry a lot when it hurts. Thank God it doesn't hurt everyday, just some days for no reason.

This morning I went to the Park da Estefanea, looking for my friends the actors, but they were gone except for two girls I recognized. They were now mostly strangers and they had another director. She was very bossy and I could no longer be a director. I could only be an actress. I didn't care for that, so I returned to reading books at another park because the ones left there I already had read or were boring.

Papa has kept his promise. Whenever he has a trip out of town, he takes me with him on his *lambretta*. He is like a teacher, always correcting everything I do or say, and he has been teaching me how to read a map. He will pull his *lambretta* to the side of the road and say in his very heavy German accent, "Okay, Verónica look at the map and tell me where to go from this point."

I am always scared that if I mess up in the directions he will never take me with him, so I am very careful when I answer, "I believe that this map might be a little off - it looks like we should be going the other way."

"Yes," he responds, "of course, because most Portuguese maps are either outdated or they are incorrectly printed. In Germany, maps are very specific and voyagers can depend on their precise and accurate maps. Germans are perfectionists, not like the Portuguese who could learn a lot from the Germans and how to make maps that are reliable and precise."

He is always bragging about Germans being of a superior race, at least much more superior than the non-educated Portuguese. I don't like the way he comes down on my fellow Portuguese since I am Portuguese and proud of it.

What I like about these trips is that I am with Papa and not only do I get to see the countryside but I get to hug him while I hold on to dear life when we travel over bumps and holes and between cars and up hills and down valleys. He stops at different towns and goes inside business buildings carrying two large cases of magazines, one in each hand. My job is to keep an eye on his *lambretta*.

On the last trip to Sacavém, a little town not too far from Lisbon, I was waiting for Papa, standing with my back against the building wall and trying to stay cool in the shade, when two old men came walking along the sidewalk. One stopped, looked at me and said to the other, "Isn't she a lovely little girl?"

He walked over to me and squeezed my nose, twisting it between his two fat fingers. He didn't count on my nose being ready to be squeezed. I had been wiping it off on my sleeves and now here it was somebody's fingers to blow off all the road dust from my nostrils. I was smiling when he found his fingers covered with snots from my runny nose. He will never again think it's cute to squeeze kid's noses.

I wish I could come up with a natural way of stopping Mama from doing something that is just as bad as the old man squeezing my nose. Just before we enter my cousin or aunt or some family or friend's house, she has the bad habit of slapping me on both cheeks to give me a rosy healthy look, and then to top it off she spits on her fingers to smooth down my eyebrows.

"Look everybody. Doesn't Verónica look so healthy! And such healthy pink cheeks!"

Well, how about mentioning the smelly lipstick spit on my eyebrows!

Max-Leão is going to marry a blonde girl some day. Every time he puts his mind to something he does just that, that's how I know. We were sitting at the community center watching a children's show on stage and there was a blonde girl sitting in front of us. He kept staring at her.

"Verónica, look isn't she beautiful with blonde hair? Some day I will marry a blonde girl!"

He said it very sure of himself, and that's how I know it's going to happen.

Mama likes me to massage her feet but I don't like to because they smell funny, and besides, feet are dirty and gross to touch unless they are my own. She has an ugly scar that goes around the bottom of her right foot. When she was about five years old, she climbed on top of a closet in the back storage room of her family's grocery store, but lost her balance when she was reaching for a large glass container full of cookies. When she fell, the bottom of her foot got cut on the broken glass. The whole bottom of her foot was sliced off and laying on the floor when her father — hearing her screaming — came to her rescue. Where they lived in Brazil there were no hospitals, but her father was a very smart man and he immediately got some honey and used it to glue the bottom of her foot back on and bandaged it together with a strip of burlap material. A few days later it had healed, but it had left a scar. Mama is very proud of her father's ingenuity and how it saved her foot. I can't even imagine Mama being a naughty kid.

Winter of 1955

Cousin Esther has been caught drinking vinegar. Someone told her that drinking vinegar helps to lose weight, and she wants to maintain her slim waist. Vinegar has been banned from Aunt Heydee's apartment, but no one can stop Esther from buying it at the grocery store and drinking a bottle before she even reaches home. It sure works; she is beautiful. She has a slim little waist and big boobs, which show well when they stick out from her low cut blouses. She looks like the movie star Marilyn Monroe. Men go crazy when they see Esther walking in the streets. Every time we go out we get a flock of half a dozen of them following us like lost dogs.

I had a lot of dogs following me home when we stayed at Costa da Caparica this summer. Every time I saw a stray dog, I kind of conned him into following me by whistling at him, then another one would appear at a street corner, then another, and sometimes I would get home with about three or four dogs. I bragged to the family about the dogs following me as if I had some kind of magic power, but I stopped when Max-Leão made fun of me and said I probably smelled like a dog and that's why I was being followed.

For *Carnaval*, Mama got me a cowboy costume. A blue cowboy hat to match the silky blue pants and jacket rented from a real costume shop. We all went to Grandma's house for pictures. Grandma Rica no longer lives there but Aunt Heydee, Aunt Ligia, and Aunt Morena do, and somehow Grandma Rica is still there in spirit.

Papa says that when you are loved you don't really die; you continue to live in the hearts of the beloved ones.

I don't agree with him, for living is feeling and Grandma Rica doesn't feel anymore, I know that, because I have seen her stone in the cemetery. Maybe what Papa means to say is that she lives as a memory, like pictures are memories, and sometimes they can live longer than people.

Uncle Augusto had fun taking our picture and when he asked me to create a pose I pointed my cowboy gun at cousin Leão, who I hate.

I really like cousin Esther, because she is fun to be with and we get to talk about all kinds of stuff. She talks to me as if I was her own age. The only thing that bothers me is what happened last Sunday — we were lying down in her bed talking and trying to stay warm under the blankets. In the wintertime it's almost as cold inside as it is outside, and just because there's no rain or cold wind blowing through the house, it's still very cold. Unless someone has a fire going, like Encarnação does in her living room, or like Papa who uses a kerosene-heating unit when he brings paper work to do at home over the weekend. Nobody is allowed to use Papa's heater except Papa. He is the only one who knows how to light it up properly. It gets nice and warm in the room he works in but I stay away from it because sometimes he farts really badly. He asks me to sit in one of the chairs and study. I don't want to sit in a heated room warmed up by farts and heat. I can't breathe. I'd rather walk outside and freeze to death in the cold.

So cousin Esther and I were lying down under the blankets and talking about stuff in general and then she told me about our cousin Marcus, the lawyer. She is in love with him and he really knows how to kiss her. He takes her on trips to the country in his car and he touches her "down there" and makes her feel good. She hopes that someday he will marry her even though all the family is against the idea. He is fifty-eight years old and she is only eighteen.

Then she told me to put a finger in my vagina and play with it, like she was doing to herself. She would not talk to me while she was doing that. She was busy moaning instead. I didn't have the courage to tell her that I was confused about the situation. I didn't want to hurt her feelings and decided to imitate her moaning sounds too. I was wondering what was next. Then she suddenly stopped and said, "Wasn't it wonderful? Did you enjoy it, too?"

I said, "Yes, of course." And I looked away afraid that she could tell that I was lying.

"This is our little secret," she said, "you are not to tell anyone."

I agreed wholeheartedly.

Max-Leão is so lucky; he had dinner with the porters downstairs. I have always wondered what the porters' house looks like on the inside. When they talk to me or anyone else they always stand by the door half closed behind them so you really can't look inside. Because they are very short, I imagine they have very small rooms with very small furniture like the small people in Gulliver's Travels.

Max-Leão told us that their place is nicer than ours. He also said that the porter made a lot of noise while slurping the hot soup from his spoon, and so did his wife and their son.

I couldn't believe it! But I guess that's the way it is when you are not well educated in the manners of social life. If Encarnação had not shown me how to eat properly a few years ago when I was having lunch with her, I would be slurping too and also chewing the food with my mouth open.

Max-Leão and I have a lot of fun sticking bubble gum into the doorbells and running away. We always ring the bell to the top floor because this way they can't catch us. It takes a while to get down the steps, and that gives us time to run away. The people have to come downstairs and pull the gum out if they want the bell to stop ringing.

Spring of 1955

I have been placed into a semi-private class for math and Portuguese grammar at the home of two old retired teachers. We are about eight kids of all ages, and we sit at a long wide table and get tested every day. I don't know anyone so I don't talk to anybody. I try to do my work and that's all. One of the teachers gets really bothered by my hairstyle and keeps coming up to me and pulling the hair off my face. She doesn't believe that I can see anything that way. She doesn't know that I cover my face purposely so that I can feel invisible. Mama thinks that I am trying to look like Veronica Lake, the American movie star. But I am not; besides she is an adult and I am still a kid. I just like hiding from everybody, so that I don't really exist. I enjoy being in my own miserable and lonely world. I don't talk to anybody, and I walk alone. Mama doesn't let me have friends and I don't need them either.

As I left the tutoring house one of the sisters was rubbing Vaseline on her hands, and she was explaining to one of the mothers picking up her daughter that Vaseline kept her hands soft and young. I wonder why she doesn't use the Vaseline all over.

Summer of 1955

Cousin Esther was handcuffed and taken to jail this weekend. Two policemen were scouting the beach of Estoril and took her in for indecent exposure. I was there when it happened. She was wearing a two-piece bathing suit that only showed a little bit of her midriff, and even the leg length was longer than my shorts. When cousin Esther puts on a bathing suit it becomes automatically indecent because she is very sexy. If she lived in America she would be a sexy movie star.

It has become a summer tradition since last year for Papa to give us thirty *escudos* and Max-Leão and I run all the way to the ice cream factory just one block away from the Cesário Verde Park. When we get there we hand them our small tin cooking pot and they fill it up with strawberry ice cream. José doesn't come with us, because he can't run. Max- Leão and I take turns holding the pot filled to the brim with strawberry ice cream as we run back as fast as we can so it doesn't melt too much. When we get home, Mama divides the ice cream between all of us. Mama and Papa get larger amounts because they are bigger than us, and we kids get a large tablespoon each. This is the most delicious ice cream in the world, even better than the sorbet they sell in the streets. I eat it really slowly and I let it melt in my mouth little by little, so I can taste it longer. Besides, if I put a big spoonful in my mouth it's not only going to be gone in one gulp but my teeth will hurt from the cold.

I don't like water with ice either; I tried it the other day at a coffee shop. I asked for a glass of water and they put ice cubes in the water. I had never had ice in water before. The water was too cold and froze my tongue and throat and hurt my teeth, and I could not taste the water. I threw the ice out and then drank the water. I was really thirsty. I don't like icy water, but I do like ice by itself to chew on because it's like chewing on crunchy glass, except it's safe. I like to feel it as it melts in my mouth, going back and forth from one cheek to the other.

This summer we are not staying at the mud hut in Costa da Caparica. We are going to spend the two summer months on the second floor of a modern building in Eiriceira, which is a very small fishing village north of Lisbon. It has a shower in the bathroom! The other place only had a washing basin and we had to shower at the beach. Living here is almost like being in Lisbon in our apartment, and it even came furnished. We have to walk a bit to get to the beach, but I like it because I am allowed to play with other kids my own age and it's easy to make friends because there are so many kids and the beach is very small, everybody knows everybody. Every day I play volleyball and soccer and hang out with another girl my age. Her name is Madalena and she has beautiful small feet. Her toes are short and stubby, not long like mine, which causes a problem finding my shoe size. I have a lot of calluses from wearing shoes because they are always too stiff and tight. I told Madalena all about Grandma Rica, but I was too ashamed to tell her that I had killed Grandma with a death wish.

My favorite time of the day is during low tide when the ocean offers ponds of water within itself. I get to splash from pond to pond but I have to be careful, because without much warning the high tide comes in, and it's a long way back to the shore. I almost drowned a few days ago. I was saved by Madalena's father who happened to be by the shoreline and literally pulled me out by the hair. He is a math teacher and Mama hired him to tutor my brothers and me at home when we get back to Lisbon. Mama is now wearing a whistle around her neck and she enjoys being called "the crazy mother." She uses the whistle to find us. She tells everyone that José is her heart, Max-Leão is her soul, and I am her blood. What a dramatic statement. Everything is a drama with Mama. Papa says it's because she was born in Brazil.

Mama has been sowing a bathing suit for Manuel, a friend of my brothers. She says Manuel's family can't afford to buy him a bathing suit; they are even poorer than us.

I don't like Manuel because he told me that he had seen me naked the other day when I was changing into my bathing suit inside the *cabana,* consequently I should be his girlfriend since he already saw me nude.

That has to be a lie because I always pull the *cabana*'s front cover strings nice and tight so that no one can see me while I change my clothes; therefore he had to be spying. I don't like him. He rubs me the wrong way by making a fib. He acts like he has one over me, and he follows me around. I told him to get lost. I feel embarrassed when he looks at me. Maybe he did see me naked. What a horrible thought. I hate him. I told Mama about Manuel but she defended him, saying he is just a kid and most likely he said that because he likes me. But I don't like him, and he had better like someone else instead of me.

This morning was one of the most embarrassing days in my life. My beach friends and I were sitting and talking behind the cabanas, up on one of the sandy hills, when Mama found us. She was laughing and being friendly with all of them and then she proceeded to teach them the Brazilian game of kissing. My own mother, whom I cannot recall ever playing with us, suddenly turned into the best buddy anyone can wish for. My friends were impressed with her when she had a boy and a girl sitting back to back and each would turn their head sideways, if they turned it to the same side they would have to kiss each other. I was horrified. The idea of kissing a boy that I don't like, like Manuel, is plain disgusting to me. I think Mama is crazy. Some of the kids got all excited about the game and they were willing to try it. I left when it came close to my turn to sit back-to-back with some icky pimple-faced boy.

While I was treasure hunting for seashells, I fell down on some green rocks by the ocean. The green was slippery slime, so I found out. I cried from the back pain and my legs felt paralyzed afterwards. It was very scary and it took awhile before I could get up and walk again.

Autumn of 1955

Max-Leão and I were walking home from playing at the park and he found a couple of odd-looking balloons on the street corner down from our house. Why people throw away perfectly good balloons is beyond us. He gave me one balloon and we filled them up with water the best we could, and took turns spraying at each other. We also like to blow them big to see how far they can stretch. Max-Leão is greedy he has more than one balloon but he doesn't want to share them with me, so I have to go out to find my own. Max-Leão is very lucky indeed; he even finds coins around park benches. It never fails, every time we go out he will find at least one *centavo*. I have no luck. I have never found any money and now I got into trouble because Mama found a used balloon in my skirt pocket. Mama was very upset and said if she ever finds out that we are picking balloons from the street like gypsy beggars, we will be beaten so bad that they will have to take us to the hospital.

I told her that they were perfectly good balloons and they didn't even have holes. She told us that they are not real balloons. They are rubber balloons used for spitting by street drunks with disgusting contagious lung diseases. Max-Leão and I were totally grossed out by what she told us and we will never again pick rubber balloons from the streets, that's for sure.

Papa is still working hard at selling magazines and butter door-to-door but we are doing okay with what we have. Max-Leão has become lazy and is not doing well in school. José is always sick and Mama's health is also bad. Papa says that I am his miracle since I am the only one that is healthy and without problems. I guess he doesn't know that my bones hurt a lot every once in awhile.

Aunt Heydee comes over to help me with household chores, which is great because I have to do the washing on the large stone basin where I used to bathe with my brothers when we were kids. After washing and beating the clothes onto the stone ridges and twisting the water out I have to hang the bed sheets and all the other clothing on the ropes outside our sunroom window. After the wash gets dried I have to stretch everything and sprinkle it with water to get some moisture back before I iron the towels and bed sheets. Papa's shirts have to be ironed with starch, and the pants have to be cleaned and brushed with soap and water and aligned just right to get the crease in the right place. I feel like Cinderella. We both have a lot in common when it comes to working like an animal all day. It takes hours to iron the bed sheets and towels and the worst is the starching of Papa's shirts. I burned my left wrist yesterday ironing one of his shirts because the light is not strong enough in the kitchen and once it's dark outside the room is gloomy too. The iron is an old clunker that has to be heated up first until the coal is burning just right. It is a very heavy iron.

I hate waxing the floors once a month and, oh yes, dusting. That is what I hate the most: dusting.

I am sick again. I caught a very bad cold. Mama told Papa that I got sick because I have weak lungs and doing this kind of housework can actually kill me. A part-time maid was hired again. Cooking over the stove is still something that they don't expect me to do; the little stove we cook on is not safe for me to handle since I am a child. Mama asked me to make a lettuce salad and when I brought it to the table she reprimanded me for not cutting the leaves into smaller, bite-sizes.

"What are we, rabbits?" she asked me.

"No, we are not rabbits," I responded trying to control my tears, "but this is my very first salad and no one showed me how small the leaves are to be cut."

Without any sympathy she said, "Now you know! Take the salad back to the kitchen and cut the pieces smaller."

When I am not working like a slave, I read. During naptime I always wander into the next park to read their library books or visit Encarnação to read her oversized African books. Thank God for books, and most of all thank God for my friend Encarnação!

How I love Aunt Heydee's cooking! She cooks the best food in the world. When she comes over to visit us, she rarely eats our food. She lives on what she makes from teaching French and piano lessons. She pays her bills and rent and is totally independent from everyone. She keeps her personal groceries in one of our kitchen drawers. She has a lot of pride and does everything not to be a burden to anyone. She considers having a room in our house, free to use whenever she comes over, a very special treat from my parents.

Aunt Heydee's meals are simple and tasty. My favorite is eggs and tomato. She fries minced fresh garlic in olive oil, and then she puts fresh sliced tomatoes in and lets it all cook until it turns into a brown paste. After that she adds two beaten eggs and with a wooden spoon she mixes it up until it has the right consistency. Served with a sliced boiled potato on the side, and a sprig of fresh parsley on the side, it sure is an incredibly tasty meal. Grandma's old apartment is her house and she shares it with her sister Ligia and her son Haim. I like visiting Aunt Heydee because her house always smells of fresh parsley, thyme, basil and flowers. She always has a bouquet of fresh flowers in the dining room next to her sewing machine.

At Uncle Augusto's request, Mama took me to the eye doctor. They had me read some letters from a wall chart and the eye doctor said loudly to one of his colleagues as he threw his arms in the air, "That girl is blind as a bat." Then he came over to Mama and reinforced his opinion once again, giving her a piece of paper and saying, "You better get this prescription filled as soon as you can; your daughter is basically blind."

He was nasty and crude like all doctors are. I hate doctors except Uncle Augusto. He would never say something like that in front of me; he would have taken Mama to the side and then tell her privately, "Verónica is blind as a bat."

I don't believe that I am blind, because I can see everybody around me. This thing about being blind is complete news to me. This has got to be payback, I already know. I used to tease some of the kids around our neighborhood, calling them "four-eyes" because they wore glasses, and now it's my turn to be made fun of. The eyeglasses will be ready at the end of the month. I don't intend to use them. I can see perfectly without them.

I like it when I am sick. Mama always treats me kindly when I am not well. She went to a lunch party and brought me a little piece of turkey. "This was all I could hide in the paper napkin inside my pocketbook," she said as she handed me the tasty morsel. I had never had turkey before. It was a little drier than chicken, but tasty. Mama was thinking about me. She must love me after all. The truth is that I don't know if she really loves me, but at moments like this when she carries a piece of turkey all the way home just for me, it makes me believe that she does love me, somehow. She is not as affectionate towards me as she is towards my brothers. I wish that she would kiss and hug me like she does my brothers. Maybe she brought the turkey piece out of pity for her sick, dying child.

Wow! I am blind! I can't believe how much better I can see with glasses. Everything is brighter and I can see so much better from far away, like across the street I can see people's faces, if they are smiling or just going on with their own business. I love it! It's like having binoculars. But Mama hates it! I am not to use glasses when we go out together. As a matter of a fact glasses make me so ugly that I'm not to use them when visiting family with her. It must embarrass her that I am almost blind. I'm allowed to use them only when I really need them, like when I am alone or when I go back to school someday.

Winter of 1956

José and I were alone at home and lying in our parents' bed. They have the softest and thickest blankets. It was cold and we decided to get under the blankets and keep warm. Naturally, trying to stay warm under the covers, we cuddled up to each other really close. It felt good being so close to him, but it scared me because he is my brother and not my boyfriend. I immediately got up and said that I was warm enough. I can never tell this to anyone. I don't believe that José was aware of what happened to me. I would die if he did.

Mama hired the rabbi to come to our house to teach Max-Leão and I to read Hebrew. Papa refuses to go to the temple, he doesn't believe in religion, he says it's all man-made, a way to control the ignorant masses. There aren't many Jews left in Portugal. "Everybody is getting old," Mama says, "and dying, and the younger ones are either getting married with *goims* or leaving to other countries where there's a chance to have a future and a better life."

Max-Leão will be having his *bar mitzvah* when he turns thirteen years old. He has to learn Hebrew whether he likes it or not. To me, the Hebrew language is as hard to understand as math! The rabbi wants us to learn the alphabet like parrots, but first I need to know what each letter means. This is like learning Greek or Chinese; it makes no sense to me. He wants us to memorize it first, but I can't. I can't even memorize a poem. I can't even remember the words to a tune. I was born with a lousy memory. And to make it worse, the rabbi falls asleep while he is teaching us which can only prove that he is as bored as we are, since he is seated and not laying down. I can never sleep sitting up, I need a pillow and a bed.

Max-Leão was trying to kick me under the table, and hit the rabbi's shin instead. The rabbi woke up angry, rubbing his injured knee. The rabbi wanted to know who did it. Max-Leão pointed to me, and he believed him! So, when the rabbi started to doze off again, I kicked as hard as I could under the table, trying to get Max-Leão back, but once again the rabbi's leg was in the way. He was furious and complained to Mama and now I don't have to learn Hebrew, only Max-Leão has to do it. It serves him right for getting me into trouble that he started!

A few days ago Mama sent me out to the corner store on an errand. I was closing the front door to the street when the grocery boy that had just delivered our groceries was also coming out of the building from the servant's door. It was raining hard and he asked me if I wanted to walk with him under his umbrella. We were both going in the same direction. I saw nothing wrong with the idea and accepted the offer. He was about my height and was very friendly in a brotherly way towards me. We talked about the rain and rubber boots, and when we got to the street corner I said goodbye and crossed the road to the bakery and he went on to the grocery store a little down the street.

This morning I got up with a fever and a cold. And then as if being sick was not enough I heard Mama telling everybody that I am sick because I am in love with the grocery boy. She saw me walking down the street under his umbrella. This really makes me mad, since it's not true. I am not in love with him or anyone else. This is totally stupid and I could scream with anger at these false accusations.

I was lying down on the old, falling-apart, green couch, and I began picking the lose strings that were just begging to be pulled off. I know this makes Mama very upset, but what the heck I was bored and the fever kept me laying there without anything to do but stare at the ceiling. So I picked one string carefully. The idea was to pull one string and see if I could out-do the next one to be longer than the first. The problem came as to where to hide them. With each string I pulled off, I rolled it with my fingers into a little ball and put it in my ears, and then my nose and finally running out of holes, I put them into my vagina. It seemed to me to be a good hiding place to put the strings. My plan was to get rid of the evidence when no one was looking. But Mama must have been watching me from the half-closed door, because she came in all upset — not because I was pulling the couch's strings, but because I was putting them in my vagina.

She said I was a nasty girl and that I was playing with myself.

I kept telling her that I was bored and there was nothing else to do but pull the couch's strings. I showed her the strings coming out of my ears and my nose so that she would not be mad at me, but she would not believe me.

She said that I was probably thinking about the grocery boy. What the heck is she talking about? I have no idea.

Mama is more messed up in the head than I thought to be possible. She took me into the bathroom this morning asked me to sit down on a chair and open my legs, because she was making an inspection of my vagina.

I cried and cried and begged her not to do that to me but she would not listen and forced me to sit there like a nincompoop with my legs opened while she kept saying, "Keep your head up and stop trying to see what I am doing." Then she presented to me, pinched by her own personal eyebrow tweezers, a caterpillar worm. "Here," she said, acting as if she had just found the worm inside of me, "you have worms growing in your vagina, because of playing with yourself yesterday."

137

I started laughing, "Mama, I was only storing the strings." I said, "This is crazy, I know it's not true what you are saying, you got those creatures from our backyard!"

"Are you calling me a liar?" she said indignantly.

"No," I said, giving up, "You are right. I was playing with my vagina, that's why I have worms growing inside of me." And I started to cry, I was afraid that she might beat me up if I didn't go along. It takes so little to please people, just lie and go along with whatever they want, it's the only way they will leave you alone.

Mama always has something to say that makes me feel guilty. Papa rarely talks to us, he is too busy working to show any interest in our lives. He works and gives all his money to Mama. Papa never says anything to make me feel bad; for that reason I tend to appreciate him more than Mama. She knelt next to my bed last night and asked me, "Verónica, who do you love more, your father or me?"

With my fingers crossed, I answered, "You, of course." But she got angry.

"You are lying," she said, "You love your father more than me." And she left the bedroom.

I wondered how she knew. I cried myself to sleep.

I lost my front tooth! Max-Leão, José and I were playing in my bedroom veranda facing the street and they decided to play the game "squeezing oil," which is a boy's game, a real stupid game. The idea is for everybody to grab one person and squeeze that person against the wall, as hard as you can. They ganged up on me, squeezing me against the wall, and then I got a good turn at squeezing Max-Leão with José helping me, but Max-Leão squeezed himself out and I fell forward into the cement wall, hitting my mouth into the corner of the brick wall. My front tooth came out, root and all. We were all screaming, seeing blood all over and Mama came running, and after washing my face there I was, crying, toothless.

After I finish chewing "Chiclets," my favorite gum, I stick it between my two front teeth and, even though I no longer smile, at least I know that there's no empty space when I talk. Mama took me with her to visit Encarnação a few days ago and I sat next to her, keeping my mouth closed, trying to nod at everything. Eduardo, her son, came in and asked what was wrong with me.

Mama said, "Oh, she is shy because she lost one of her baby teeth but it will grow back soon."

Everybody was surprised about her comment, including Eduardo, who immediately asked, "She is still losing baby teeth at almost twelve years old? Isn't that kind of late?"

Mama was ready with an the answer. "Yes, but this is the last one, if you look up close you will see that there's a little white piece starting to stick out, her new tooth — just about breaking through."

So, there I was with my mouth wide open so that Eduardo, Encarnação, and her cousin Carlos, the accountant could take turns at admiring the tip of my new tooth. Mama knows very well that the white is just an imaginary thing, since they were all staring at my gum and nothing else. How Mama gets away with her stories is beyond me.

"How long will it take for the tooth to grow completely out," they asked with curiosity.

"Hmm," Mama took a few moments to come up with another fib, "Hmm, according to her dentist, who is a specialist, about two more months."

Two months, I thought to myself, *this is definitely going to be a miracle. The tooth and the root are in the garbage, gone into the "La de da Tooth Land of No Return."*

I was very lucky that I didn't cut my face open or cut my lip with a huge gap, or worse. I could have been scarred for life, said Mama on the way home. Yeah, and how about punishing my two stupid brothers for pushing me into the wall? No, it's always my fault!

It's all over the radio and the news, North America has a new sound, and it's called rock and roll. The singer that can make everybody move is Elvis Presley, "The Pelvis." When he sings, nobody can stand still; even old people in wheelchairs get up to dance to his music.

~Chapter Four ~

The Enlightenment

Spring of 1956

I like sitting and listening to Mama and her sisters talking. I learn a lot that way, and I am so quiet that I believe that for the most part they don't even know that I am there. I have learned that *goims* have different penises than Jews. *Goims* have a skin hanging out on the tip of it and a lot of them are not very clean and give infections to their wives. I don't dare ask how that happens, but I heard Aunt Heydee tell Mama that one of her piano students likes that her husband has extra skin hanging out, because it gives longer pleasure while having sex.

I'm starting to realize that sex must have something to do with rubbing the penis against the vagina and also putting it inside, but at the same time I can't even imagine such a thing. It must hurt like hell.

I can smile again. Aunt Heydee took me to her dentist. He likes her a lot, and because of that, he gave her a special discount price to take a mold of my teeth and build me a tooth on a little pink transparent plastic plate, which sticks to the roof of my mouth with a touch of dental cement. At night before I go to sleep, I scrub the tooth and the plate attached to it with a toothbrush and soap and soak it overnight in a glass with water. This gives me time to recover, because the roof of my mouth is very sore and red. I am allergic to the plastic.

I am never going to get used to Mama's cooking. I was getting yelled at for not eating dinner, which consisted of boiled spaghetti mixed with boiled chunks of meat, and I was trying not to breathe in the dreadful smell coming from my dish which reminded me of a dog, I mean a dirty street-dog smell. I was praying for a miracle, anything that would get me out of eating the food in front of me, when we heard the screeching sound of brakes coming from the street accompanied by a lot of screaming. We ran to the window, and what happened was a car hit a dog. He was lying on the ground, dead. The dog owner had grabbed the motorist and was trying to choke him for killing her dog. When we got back to the table, I wanted to throw up even more from the smell of the food. Mama was very understanding when I told her that I could not finish dinner, I had just seen a dog die. Max-Leão offered to eat my food, since he loves spaghetti. Thank God!

Cousin Esther finally got her way and married cousin Marcos, "The old goat," as everybody refers to him. He told the family that he is going to keep Esther pregnant and barefoot and in less than five years she will look as fat and old as him. Not a pretty picture.

José is so lucky! Just because he has asthma, he gets special meals, like steak and fried potatoes, while Max- Leão and I get fried liver. José gets sandwiches made with finely sliced deli meat, like ham and cheese. Max-Leão and I get bread with butter. Whenever Mama gives me money to run to the grocery store and get some meat and cheese for José's sandwiches, I always steal a slice of the delicious salty ham. I feel guilty that I am stealing food from my sick brother, and sometimes I only take half of a slice. I am afraid to get caught.

I have been practicing at making asthmatic sounds by breathing hard. Max-Leão put his ear to my chest and said it sounds real. I have become very good at it. Mama might fall for it. Max-Leão told me that if it works he would do the same. My lungs sound terrible when I take a deep breath. The wheezing can't be missed, and Mama believes that I have asthma.

My plan didn't work. Mama took me to our cousin who specializes in sick children. He was too smart for me because he asked me to clear my throat and cough before using the stethoscope on my chest. Once I coughed, I had nothing in my throat to play with. I was given a clean bill of health.

Summer of 1956

Something very strange and wonderful happened to me today, when everybody at home was taking a nap after lunch as customary, I decided instead to take a walk up to the *Fonte Luminosa*, just a few blocks from our house.

Now that I am twelve years old, I am allowed to walk in the city by myself as long as I am not too far away from home. The *Fonte Luminosa* is an inviting fountain to cool off, and I like to stare at the bigger-than-life marble statues of beautiful naked women and men on horses. From the top of the fountain, a cascade of waterfalls fills up the pool below with cool water and if I am lucky to be in the way of a breeze, the waterfall turns into a misty shower around me. I like taking my sandals off and sitting on the fountain's edge dangling my feet in the water. It feels refreshing.

Sleeping in the middle of the day is impossible for me, and this time of the day it's more like torture since I can always hear the snoring coming from my parents' bedroom. It is an irritating annoying sound. Papa sounds like a rolling train with brake trouble, and Mama whistles. Everything closes down at this time of the day and for two hours the city sleeps. This was going to be the perfect time for me to escape.

I never reached the fountain. It was hotter than I thought. As always when it gets too hot, I got a pounding headache. The sun was unmerciful, heating the top of my head to feel like a bursting volcano. I could barely see except through the slits of my eyes as I squinted through the unbearable sunlight, trying to see the street pavement below my feet. The further I walked, the more my hands got puffy and stiff, and I could hardly close them. There was no shade; just long stretches of cobblestone streets. I kept thinking that I should turn around and go back home, but like Mama says, I am hard-headed and once I put my mind to something there's no turning back. The heat from a broken-down brick wall showed me how hot it was when I barely rested my back against it. Nothing was living around me except a tiny salamander running up the wall.

Beyond the tall wall and through the cracks and holes I tried to see what was on the other side. Except for some spots of burned-out weeds and dried-up grass, the soil was just a huge canvas of desert ground. After a few more steps, I looked again beyond an old metal rusty door with a lock and metal chain around it which meant that it was off limits to enter. In the distance I could see a huge home that, by its neglect, must have been abandoned many years ago. It looked desolate, as if crying in the loneliness of its surroundings. *What had happened to its owner?* I wondered. Was the ground salted so that nothing could grow there, like they used to do a few years back to the enemies of the state? Perhaps a girl my age and her family had been killed for political reasons; it would not be the first time. Everybody knows that our president Salazar, is a dictator and as such he is merciless against his enemies.

I looked around. Not a soul walking or a car going by; only silence and the sun burning my skin and my vision. I was thirsty and tired of walking, when I smelled roses. Not just the smell of roses, but the smell of tiny little baby roses. There it was, one wild little pink button-rose escaping from

I Found God Today!

the dead garden and squeezing itself through the cracked wall and peeking out into the world outside. A few steps down where part of the wall had fallen, the same rosebush was sprouting all over, covering the ugly wall and screaming how beautiful life is. I stayed there next to it, taking one deep breath after another and immersing myself in the scent. There was a complete sense of being; the sense of what it feels like to have God all around. I laughed and screamed from outside inwards. The sound of silence was loud and clear within me, and the feeling was joy to my soul, running through my skin and inwards again, from my eyes and from my mouth and lungs. I was breathing in life.

I am not telling anyone about this; no one would believe me, and they would think that I am a sissy. This is my secret, my very intimate secret; I no longer have to look for God in a temple, or in a church, or any specific place, because God is everywhere. I will never be alone again.

We are back for the summer at Costa da Caparica, but I don't really care for this beach anymore. It's too big and lonely. I would rather be in Eiriceira with my friend Madalena.

Mama gave me a big speech about walking around the house in my bathing suit when Papa is home for the weekend. She said that a bathing suit is not the proper attire to use at home; it is indecent to walk around half-naked. Just because Papa is my father he is still a man.

I get hurt when she says things like that; she makes me feel ashamed of my body and being a girl. I wish I was a boy like my brothers, and then perhaps I could be closer to my parents, without all these bizarre innuendos.

Summertime can be very boring. It's been very, very hot and muggy and it's hard to do anything but be immersed in the ocean for hours. The shade is no help. I was sitting on the sidewalk with my brothers and a few of his friends passing the time talking and they gave me a cigarette to try. All Americans and British smoke, because they are fashionable

146

and educated. We see that in foreign movies too, it's very "cool" and chic to smoke. I was dying to try it. I took a puff and choked on the smoke. I didn't like it, but I didn't want to say anything. I didn't want to offend the kids I was hanging out with, so I held the cigarette in my hand and pretended that I was puffing away. I would have felt more appropriate if I had a chimney on top of my head. When I tried to breathe in and out to make little circles of smoke like they did, the smoke went in the wrong pipe and I couldn't breathe, very much like drowning in smoke instead of water. I didn't like it at all, and then to make it more embarrassing, an old man went by and criticized me with a disgusted look in his eyes. "It's disgraceful to see a pretty young girl smoking like a man."

Everybody made fun of the old man going by, calling him "old fart." I threw my cigarette away.

Maria, our part-time maid became friendly with a fisherman that owns one of the giant half moon shaped fishing rowboats boats, and she offered to take my brothers and me on a trip to the sea this morning. We all sat at the tip of the boat, the highest spot. I was very excited about my fishing adventure. But what I didn't expect were the tall waves that made the boat feel like it was going to turn over. It went up and down like a roller coaster. I screamed and screamed and told them I was going to throw up and I wanted to go back to the shore. When I threw up all over, they turned the boat back to shore and left me there, after calling me names and yelling at me, as if it was my fault that I have a weak stomach. I was shaking, and it took me a while before I felt normal again.

Papa is still selling butter door-to-door. The gold glass with the lady's face engraved on it is always in and out of the pawnshop along with the diamond moon-shaped pin with thirty-five diamonds that Grandpa Leão bought for Grandma Rica when they were still rich. It belonged to the last queen of Portugal. These two items have saved us various times when we are having a drop on finances. Papa has been selling a lot more books and magazines to architects and foreigners, and that is why we can afford to come here for the summer. Still, we only see Papa on weekends. He still drives his Lambretta, and last week he told me that one-day when he can afford a new one, he will show me how to drive it and will give it to me. I didn't tell him that I am afraid of driving a motorcycle; I have never even driven a bike. He always thinks that I am able to do anything, but he is wrong. I am a *medricas*, which means that I am a "scaredy-cat" when it comes to possibly getting hurt.

I hang out with Max-Leão and José all day like Mama wants me to, but I have not told her that we play with *goims*, and I use my glasses so that I can see better. We are all buddies and take long walks through the woods and have been trying to find a nude beach that's supposed to be only a few miles south of us, but no matter how much we walk we never seem to find it.

These last few days have been very, very hot, and I have stopped going out with them. I get sick with a pounding headache from the sun. If the boys want to do that, they can go by themselves. I feel funny being the only girl in the group anyway, and besides I don't need to look at naked people. I already know women have a vagina and two breasts, men have a penis and no breasts, and everybody has a butt, some bigger than others. What's the big deal?

I had to fight for my honor today! Max-Leão told me that one of the boys in our group was passing the word around that I had kissed him and that I was his girl. I went out looking for him. Costa da Caparica is not that big, the beach is enormous but the town is less than an hour to tour. There he was, the scoundrel, the liar, sitting on a bar stool at the local tavern, most likely telling the bartender about me. I walked up to him, made a closed fist and without a single word I punched him in the face with all my mighty force. He didn't even know what hit him. It was that quick, and he was

on the ground on his back with a bloody lip and holding his
face as I walked out, proud of myself.

I saw him a few times in town and he always walks away
from me. There have been a lot of mixed opinions. Some
said he got what he deserved, others said I was not very lady-
like and I should have talked to him instead. I am too shy to
do that and I can't deal with confrontations. In the back of
my mind I wonder if the whole thing was not a lie, maybe he
was innocent, and I had punched the wrong person.

Aunt Heydee said that if I accuse an innocent person of a
crime, I am guilty of that sin myself and I must be very
careful before I point the finger, or God will punish me for it.
From now on I promise never to jump to conclusions until I
know for sure that what someone tells me about someone
else is true.

We spend a lot of our time at the coffee house in the main
street in Costa da Caparica. Mama likes to sit there with
company like aunts Heydee, Morena or Ligia, when they
come over on weekends and we sit under the large outside
umbrella shade, each sipping a cup of coffee that lasts all
afternoon. I usually have mine with lots of milk added to it
because coffee makes me jittery, and my hands shake like
those of an old lady. We sit looking at all the tourists going
by and there's always some kind of gossip going on.
Sometimes I can't believe my own ears.

"Did you see the way our young cousin Joseph was
holding Alexandra by the waist while teaching her to roller
skate?"

And the other would say, "She is married but I bet you
that on the way back to Lisbon while on the bus they really
got closer to each other."

"Well, can you blame her; he is very handsome. I bet
they went straight from the bus into his bed."

Gossip is very entertaining and it helps to pass the idle
time we have hanging out at the coffee shops during the long
and hot afternoons.

Television is a new household item. It is so new that no one can afford it, except coffee shops and tavern owners who use it to entice customers to shop and spend long hours in their establishment. The only person I know that has a television at home is Encarnação, but she is not very rich, just well-to-do with her monthly pension. She also lends money to Mama every once in awhile when Papa is not making enough to pay the rent or buy food, and so on.

Our favorite coffee shop is situated in the center of Costa da Caparica. The owner will always have more customers than the other coffee house down the street because he has a television for the customers to look at; therefore this is the place to catch all the news from the outside world. For a couple of months now, Papa has been trying to sell colored filters to television owners. Basically the filter is nothing but a colored plastic sheet; a see-through plastic film with three basic colors. The bottom is green, the middle is brownish red and the top is blue for the sky. That is supposed to make the black and white television look like color television. The film is also supposed to stick to the television screen but most of the time it slides off. It is the latest in technology from Germany. Papa gave the coffee shop owner a colored filter, in the hopes that it will serve as an advertisement and someone will want to buy one for their black and white television. But no one at Costa da Caparica has inquired about buying a filter from Papa. I really don't believe that Papa is going to do well with these colored television filters. People here are very poor and don't have a television, and that's why they come to the coffee shop to see the news. Papa is also selling German perfume, a special perfume that is supposed to take headaches away when rubbed gently on the temples. I tried, but the smell gave me a headache.

I am in love! Of course he doesn't know that I love him; I would rather die than let him know it. His name is João and he is one of Max-Leão's friends. He is slim, and taller than me, has dark hair, and beautiful almond-shaped brown eyes. He is one year older than I am. We all go out together during the day but we rarely say anything. We just stare at each other, because we are both shy. Saturday night I was in my bed reading a murder mystery book when a small stone hit my bedroom window. It was João and two other friends asking if both my brothers and I would like to go out with them. My heart almost jumped out of my chest.

I only see João during the day; I am not allowed to go out at night. So, Max-Leão and José went out with the boys and I stayed home. I tried to read my book, but I couldn't concentrate. I wanted to go out too, and have some fun with our friends. I feel so sad. I feel so lonely and sad.

João commented on my white blouse this afternoon because it has seashells all around the top. This is my favorite shirt and I wear it every day with my green shorts. I know that this shirt makes me look the best I can look. Mama made it for me, and of all the clothes she made, this is a masterpiece of design. It's not too big or too tight, it's my size and it's made of white cotton, and it goes well with anything I want to wear. Anyway, João was looking at me and said, smiling, "You have nice seashells."

I didn't know what to say. I just smiled back. I know he likes me too; he might even love me.

We are going back to Lisbon in two weeks, it's the end of the summer, and most likely we will never see each other again. After all, he is a *goim*. Love is so painful. I wish him the best. I will think of him every day from now on and imagine being in his arms as he holds me tenderly and kisses me passionately, just like in the American movies.

Summer is almost over. It's already getting cooler at night. Running around in the water, walking on the sand as far as my feet can take me, laying in the sun all day, playing "nail" with my brothers, long walks in the afternoon, reading, and listening to Mama and my aunts gossiping at the café; will be old history soon.

"Did you see what happened to that young couple on their honeymoon? They had to leave after a week of too much sex, swimming, and staying up all night, not necessarily in that order." They were laughing heartily.

"Yes," one of my aunts agreed, "poor girl; she got really sick, probably anemia and he had some kind of a virus. Who knows what they both wound up with? A honeymoon can make you seriously ill, even kill you if you are not careful."

I can't believe this nonsense as if getting married and being happy can actually hurt you. Of course I didn't say anything, the couple was probably sickly to begin with.

Autumn of 1956

We had a fire on the sub-floor directly underneath our apartment in Lisbon. Heavy dark smoke was coming out through the windows below us. The firemen were yelling for everyone to evacuate the building immediately. Max-Leão, José and I followed Mama as she ran to her bedroom to grab her lottery ticket for the week, then we all ran out of the house. The fireman had to break the windows of the apartment below us, where the "kept woman" lives. They were yelling at Elena to open the front door, but she had locked herself in and couldn't find the key. It was horrible to hear her screaming from inside the apartment. Finally one of the firemen climbed up a ladder to her window, broke it with a hammer, and went in to get her. He carried her out in his arms as we all clapped our hands in admiration of his courage and successful mission. Everybody noticed and commented that the fireman that carried her out had a big smile on his face, because she was wearing a sexy blue dainty lacy nightgown covered by a matching silk robe.

She was taken in an ambulance because the bottom of her feet had been severely torched by the burning wooden floors. The firemen did a great job controlling the fire from spreading up into our floor or down further into the porter's apartment. Later when Elena returned from the hospital, we found out that she had the key to the front door in one of the pockets in her robe the whole time that she was screaming while burning her feet. She had panicked and forgotten where she had the key. Everybody felt that the "kept woman" deserved whatever bad happens to her because she is living off a married man and destroying his family. I don't agree. There is no good reason for anyone including a "kept woman" to get burned alive. How about the married man, how come he is looked upon as the innocent victim of her spell? Besides, Mama is the one that always says, "It takes two to Tango."

I was walking home from Encarnação's house and I almost got killed. The men working at the garage two blocks from our house were standing by their door and when they saw me they began whistling at me and one of them said, "Come here little girl, I have a doll for you." They were laughing. "What's the matter," yelled the other next to him, "Don't you believe us? Come here you cute thing!"

I started to run scared, and ran all the way home. I realize now how lucky I am that I was walking across the street instead of the sidewalk next to the garage. They could have grabbed me.

A few weeks ago, Papa explained to me what strangers do to girls my age when they offer dolls, candy, or any kind of presents.

We were having dinner all together and Mama said something about me looking older for my age. The way that I am blooming, she probably meant my breasts. I have also noticed that my body has been changing lately. I keep wondering if my breasts will grow as big as cousin Esther's.

"Soon men will start wanting to use you."

What was she trying to tell me? I looked at her perplexed.

"What do you mean, use me?" I asked curiously. Mama never says anything directly; I'm supposed to know automatically what she is referring to.

I guess that from the look on my face, Papa could tell that I really wanted to know what she was talking about and he said, "Have you noticed the way I lovingly and very

153

tenderly hug and kiss your mother? Well, these strangers have no loving feelings towards you. They don't love you. They will grab you for the fun of it and then squeeze you like a lemon until there's no juice left." And Papa squeezed the half-lemon next to his plate all over his boiled codfish.

That was enough for me. I promised myself that I would never again squeeze purple sea creatures at the beach, and most of all, I will always stay away from strangers.

Papa's sister and her husband Curt came from England to visit us for three days. Curt lost all his family in the concentration camp including his wife and children. He met Ilse for the first time when they were both hiding in England. They are very loving towards each other, holding hands when they walk the streets, and when they sit next to each other. They are even more loving than Mama and Papa are with each other. This surprises me because I always thought that the English and the Germans were a cold stiff kind of people that never show feelings or emotion.

Ilse asked Mama if she could take me to England with her, but Mama would never let that happen.

Aunt Ilse and her husband Curt took me out for ice cream, and then she gave me the bad news. She told me they found out that her two daughters had been gassed in the concentration camp. The last time she had been in Israel to play the violin in a concert she was reading the engraved names of the children killed during the war upon a stone wall and that's when she came across her own two girls' names along with the list of other children that were with them. There was no mistake. Her children's names had been taken from the books the Nazis kept so organized concerning who they had killed, how, and when.

I can't even imagine what she must have felt after so many years of hoping that maybe, just maybe, her children might still be alive, possibly taken to Russia by the Russian soldiers that had taken a lot of the camp survivors with them when the war was over.

She cried and cried as she spoke and then as she wiped her tears with a little white lace kerchief she said, "I still love Germany, my country. I have a lot to do yet, playing the violin and bringing happiness to the less fortunate in Germany."

After they left, I heard my parents talking about her. Basically she was to blame for having sent the two girls away to school in Holland when the war was going on. She should have stayed with them instead.

It's always easy to figure out a better way of doing things after it's done, and I am sure that Ilse feels the same way. She cannot change the past, she lives with it, and every note that she plays on her violin cries like her soul is being ripped open. I don't like the sound of the violin anymore.

I was sitting in the kitchen watching Aunt Heydee fry tomatoes with eggs for lunch, hoping she would share some with me as she always does, when Mama came in with two pictures of my cousins from North America.

She asked me, "Which one do you like the best?"

I thought she was just asking my opinion, and I chose Alberto who seemed to be younger and had a nice smile. Gabriel looked older and too serious for me.

She agreed with me, "Alberto is definitely the best looking of the two brothers. He is twelve years older than you, but that's okay, a woman should be a lot younger than the husband, that way he can't ever get bored with his young wife." And she added, "How would you like to marry him?"

"Are you kidding? Do you mean Aunt Nelly's son, my cousin?" I was shocked.

She picked up the pictures from the table and, walking away, she said, "Yes, him. And you better hope and pray for it, because if that happens you will be going to North America and you will be the luckiest woman in the world."

I didn't say anything, I didn't know what to think of all this. I believe she is just fantasizing like she does with so many things.

Our building is starting to show its age. The landlord is still collecting the same rent he charged in 1943. Nobody is moving out and by law the rent can't go up with their original owners or new family members living here. When the eldest dies, the younger takes over the rights to the apartment, going from father to son and from son to grandson and so on, but the rent remains the same. The problem is that the cost of living keeps going up and the landlord is getting the same rent he did some thirteen years ago. Everybody feels that all landlords are rich and too cheap to fix the buildings as they start needing a paint job and repairs. The carpet on the wooden steps has long been gone, worn out by the up-and-down traffic of the tenants. The wooden steps are still kept clean and waxed once a month by the porter's wife. The old couple continues to get a free apartment to live in, in exchange for cleaning the building. The planters died a few years back and there's only one cracked ceramic pot left on the right side of the steps with a plant stalk that has no leaves. Our building is starting to look more and more like grandma's apartment house. Our bathroom is literally decaying. The cracked mirror above the chipped sink reminds me of a Picasso painting as I see myself with two half noses. Aunt Heydee gladly painted some colorful flowers with oil paints to cover the ugly cracks and made it very artistic. It looks kind of French. She is an artist. We need a new mirror, but we can't afford a new one; besides, the landlord is the one that should replace it with all the money he gets from our rent. If I prop myself between the cracks there are flowers on my hair, otherwise it's on my face. The toilet water tank has brown water spots from leaking and the rope has to be wiggled in a certain way or it won't flush. The floor tiles are damaged and some of the stones have lifted up. The rooms need a coat of paint real bad; the walls have been peeling for some time. The old curtains in the living room that is part of the dining room have faded to a light shade of something that used to be.

I am not allowed to bring anyone home. I stopped asking a long time ago. A girlfriend can mean one of my brothers falling in love with her and then I would have to carry that on my conscience. Mama and Papa's grandchildren would be Catholic! I don't have any friends and I don't need any friends anyway. As long as I have books I don't care if I never talk to anyone either.

The wooden kitchen closets have started to rot on the inside but it came in very handy a few days ago. I came home with a huge bleeding gash along my right leg after getting cut on my neighbor's metal bike, which I wanted to try riding it. The cut was from below the knee to the ankle and I was bleeding a lot, but Josefina our part-time maid knew what to do. She scraped the rotten wood from the kitchen closets and applied it to the open bleeding wound. It worked like a cork on an open faucet. It stopped the bleeding. Mama came in at that moment and was appalled by the treatment. But Josefina swore on Mother Mary and Jesus her son that my leg would heal without a scar.

I have the worst cold of my life. It's been three miserable days of nose-dripping, coughing, and fever. I am not allowed to get out of my room except to the bathroom, right next to my bedroom. Nobody will come near me, they are all afraid of getting infected.

I am so bored. I already went through the usual ritual of looking at all the family picture albums and I've read all the books next to my bed, and the movie star magazines have been read over and over again. After taking a good look around my bedroom, I realized how drab it looks. There's no window, no street noises, no sunshine. The only sound I hear is when someone is flushing the toilet next to my bedroom, letting me know that there's life out there. Mama believes that by changing the rooms around, the house always has a new look, but I don't agree with that. It's just junky furniture moving around from one room to another.

I have decided to be a little creativè with my time today and brighten up my bedroom. I'm the only one that sleeps here, except for Aunt Heydee when she is visiting us. She gets to stay overnight, and she sleeps in my bed with me. Wintertime is my favorite time for sleeping next to Aunt Heydee, I get to curl up to her and stay warm all night.

I am going to decorate my bedroom today.

I spent the morning cutting all the pictures of movie stars from my collection of magazines, which I have collected through the last few years. I worked hard all afternoon with a bottle of glue and the movie stars "cut outs." I glued them to the beat-up bookcase and to the old armoire. I glued them to the walls. I glued them to the small side table next to my bed. I worked at it all day long. The start of a new life in decorating was opening up in front of my eyes. I carefully closed my bedroom door every time I went to the bathroom, because I didn't want anyone to see my work of art until I was finished.

American movie stars are the most beautiful; they are the most elegant and beautiful in the world. The French, English and German movie stars are okay but nothing like the American movie stars. My favorite is Audrey Hepburn even though she is from Belgium. I would like to look like her, but my bones are a lot larger than hers and even if I starved to death I could never be as thin as she is. There's Paul Newman and Susan Hayward (my favorites), Marlon Brando, Elizabeth Taylor, Marilyn Monroe, Burt Lancaster (Mama likes his muscles), Rock Hudson, Doris Day, Steve McQueen, Shirley Temple, William Holden, and Ava Gardner (Papa likes her, he says she has a beautiful neck, like a swan). I glued my favorite pictures so that anyone walking into the bedroom could not miss them, they would be greeted at first glance. The ugly ones, or the ones that are movie stars because they are probably good actors or they know someone that got them to play in the movies, like Katharine Hepburn, Charlie Chaplin, Ingrid Bergman, Fred Astaire, Joan Crawford, Edward G. Robinson, Charlton

Heston, Humphrey Bogart, and Betty Davis, I put them up as fill-ins.

It was six in the evening when I heard Mama closing the front door as she came into the house. Our front door makes a very distinct sound that cannot be mistaken by any other door opening or closing. I was literally exhausted from all the work I had done. My bedroom door opened about ten minutes later. She would have hit me if I hadn't looked so sick. She was livid with anger. I was to get a scrub and a bucket of water and remove every single glued picture, right then and there. According to her it was the most tasteless thing she had ever seen.

I cried and begged, but her decision was final. I spent the rest of the evening peeling and scrubbing the pictures off the walls and the furniture and no matter how much I coughed Mama didn't feel sorry for me.

Once in awhile Mama can be nice, but most of the time she is a witch. She hates me. I don't even remember why she hits me, half the time. A few years back, in order to protect myself from amnesia, I purposely stayed awake most of the night engraving into my memory the beating I had suffered that day. I swore to myself that I would always remember that beating, even if I already forgot why she beat me that day. I engraved into my memory, like a woodpecker does to a tree. I swore that I would remember that day for the rest of my life so that I would never feel bad for not loving her. It will always be easy to recall that day, because she hit me over the head without stopping all the way from my bedroom to the bathroom, which in those days was at the end of the house on the furthest side. I bled from my nose all over the floors and the sink where she finally grabbed me by the hair and pushed my head into the cold water. When I become a mother, my children can decorate their bedroom the way they like it, and I will listen and I will be understanding and never ever hit them.

The "kept woman's" lover not only had her apartment fixed up like new, but for Christmas he surprised her with a brand new red sports car parked right outside the front door. Everybody realized that even with her burned feet he is never going to leave Elena because he truly loves her.

Winter of 1957

I get a lot of bloody noses even when I am not getting hit across the face. Mama has taken me twice now to a doctor that has burned the inside of my nose. They call it cauterization, and it's supposed to help. I hate it! I think it's making it even more sensitive. In my opinion, my nose got damaged from getting hit all the time across my face and now getting it burned is making it worse. I feel like a boxer after being in the ring a few times.

This afternoon I got electrocuted and I found out that my brother Max-Leão is not only lazy, but he is also a coward. I went into the dining room in the dark and I was trying to find the socket on the wall to plug in a lamp so that I could read in Papa's favorite armchair. While I was feeling the wall, my two right fingers went into the socket holes. The cover had fallen off like most of the other sockets in the house. I learned what electricity feels like when it's not running on wires but through the body. I was shaking and could hardly stand up. There was nobody else at home as I ran towards Max-Leão when he came to see what I was screaming about, and when he saw me he ran into his bedroom and closed the door behind him. I went after him, opened his door, and walked towards him so that I could hold onto him. He grabbed a book from his desk and threw it at me, screaming, "Stay away from me."

One book hit me really hard on the head and I had to leave his room and go into my room cursing him for being so mean to his beloved sister and friend.

Thank God for roasted chestnuts in the winter. As long as there's a chestnut vendor on the street, I can always buy a few and hold them in my hands to stay warm. When they get cold, I eat them.

Mama is right, I'm just like Papa, hardheaded. I am like a stone, unmovable. I am getting better and better at hiding my feelings and it's working magnificently. Over the weekend I was in a musical play at the Jewish Youth Center, and when I went outside onto the back porch to pick up a pin — to hold my headpiece that kept falling — and reached into a basket with needles and pins, I stuck a pin in my right thumb. I was there trying to find something to put a stop to the bleeding when Uncle Augusto appeared on the veranda and asked me if I was ready to get on stage. Of course, he also asked me to pose for a picture and I held my hand tight behind my back and he didn't even know what happened. I felt too stupid and ashamed to tell him that I had hurt my hand. I am such a klutz.

There is a new family that moved in to our apartment complex about six months ago. They have a son about my age and he is really cute, with dark hair and dark eyes. They are renting the apartment below our next-door neighbor. He likes me I can tell, because when we see each other in the stairways he looks and smiles at me. Then, to make my wishes come true, he sent me a love-letter yesterday. He gave the letter to Teresa our maid to give to me. Teresa gave the letter to Mama. But of course I only heard about it when Mama spoke to his mother, telling her to keep Jorge her brat son away from me. I went to bed thinking about him and then out of nowhere I had this flushing feeling of pleasure coming up and filling me with happiness. Wow!! That's all I can say, because this is a real discovery about my body. My goodness, this must be what everybody is talking about. Sex!

Papa's oldest sister Friedel came from England this week to spend a few days with us. She asked me to be her guide around Lisbon, and I noticed that she was the opposite of Ilse her sister. When I suggested having some ice cream she said,

"Not in between meals; if you start eating in between meals, you will lose your appetite and that is a waste of food."

She was very proper, a blend of German and British manners. Her German attitude was very much like Papa's personality about everything. She made a few observations concerning the Portuguese being so melodramatic and how unnecessary it was to get up from their seat to leave the bus or trolley when it had not yet stopped completely. I'd never noticed that until she mentioned it. She also suggested that Mama should lower the gas on the stove once the food starts to boil, because it's a waste of energy and not cost-effective. Mama was upset about Friedel's meddling because that meant she was criticizing Mama's housewife knowledge, but I thought Friedel's idea of setting the gas lower was a good idea since it does save on gas once the food started to boil.

After Friedel returned to England, Papa said he admired his sister's intelligence and he went on to state that the difference between his sisters was very obvious: one was definitely smarter than the other. For example, when Ilse has company she spends days cooking and making food and preparing a feast, but when Friedel has a gathering she goes to work and makes arrangements to have a caterer bring in the food all done. Consequently Friedel has the most common sense in efficiency and she is the wiser of the two sisters because she doesn't waste precious time. How German can one be!

I heard that Jorge's family is moving very soon, and he is sick with a cold.

"I want to see him," I pleaded with Teresa our maid, "You have to help me. If you are my friend, you will help me. I didn't even have a chance to read my first love letter because Mama threw it away."

Teresa said, "I feel bad that I showed the letter to your mom, so okay, just don't get me into trouble by telling her anything and I will help you."

She closed the sunroom door behind her and, holding my hand she whispered, "I have an idea, just stay close to me and don't say anything."

We went downstairs through the back of the house and down into the basement, where she knocked at "his" door. "Excuse me," said Teresa with the face of a real actress as she smiled at "his" maid, "We are locked out of our house and I don't have the key to get back in, unless we use the front door. Do you mind if we go through your house? By the way, how is Jorge? I heard that he isn't feeling too good."

"His" maid let us in, saying, "Oh, he is just a pain, his mother is trying right now to give him some medicine for the cough but he is very difficult to handle. Well, you know how kids are."

My eyes were wide open, not wanting to miss anything around me. I wanted to see the man of my dreams, even if just a glimpse. I followed Teresa, taking my time with small steps behind her.

Then I heard a crying voice, "No, no, I don't want it, it tastes terrible."

I looked and there he was, Jorge dressed in blue flannel pajamas with little white bears, crying while his mother was trying to hold him down to make him swallow the spoonful of medicine. What in the world was I seeing? He was a crybaby! A weakling! I imagined him strong, courageous, and ready to fight the world with me. *The romance is over,* I told myself.

I thanked Teresa for her kindness in jeopardizing her job for me. I didn't tell her how disappointed I was.

I spent the afternoon with Cousin Esther. She invited me to her house and she made tea and gave me ginger cookies. We did lie down on her bed, but this time she didn't play with herself. She told me how happy she was being married, and that she was very jealous of her husband and she was always giving him demonstrations of how she felt so that he knew how much she loved him. She asked me to stay until he got home and she put on an act of jealousy for my benefit, so that I could see how it was done. She yelled and cried and accused him of not being at work but cheating on her instead, and then she winked one of her eyes at me.

The whole thing was truly theatrical, like Aunt Friedel would say, melodramatic. I felt sorry for Cousin Marcos. I will never do that to my husband.

~ *Chapter Five* ~

The Adjusting Period

1957-1959

Spring of 1957

Max-Leão came home yesterday and told Mama that he had
seen a trolley accident where a man crossing the street got
run over and his head had been decapitated. The man's head
got cut clean off from his body and had rolled over the
pavement and stopped at Max-Leão's feet. He acted very
upset about it and Mama forced him to take some of her own
medicine drops that are good to calm the nerves. Mama takes
a lot of medicine she gets for free from her brother and
cousins.

The problem with Max-Leão's story is that in today's
newspaper it was mentioned that a man had been hit by a
trolley at Praça de Chile, but he had suffered only minor
bruises to his legs. Max-Leão had lied. Mama said no, he has
not lied, he has a vivid imagination, and he should be praised
for his creativity. Later in the day I heard her tell Papa that
she was worried about Max-Leão and wondered if he was
suffering from hallucinations. Personally, I think he wants
attention and he got it.

A family from Africa has moved into our building, into the
downstairs empty apartment where Jorge and his family used
to live. Teresa told me that she has seen them and that their

skin color is black like coal. I have never seen a black person, except in the big books at Encarnação's house. I was curious, so I went in the backyard making believe that I was playing. I was hoping to see at least one of them. I saw the mother and two of her five daughters. They were not naked like in the pictures I had seen at Encarnação's house. Amelia, the mother's youngest daughter, is my age. We started talking and I asked her if I could touch her skin, and she smiled and let me touch her arms and hands. Her skin was soft like mine.

Amelia likes to talk to me about Angola, where she was born, and I love listening to her African stories. We are the best of friends. I am welcome to her house and today I helped Amelia's mom prepare for a party this weekend. They let me beat the eggs for a little while until they noticed that I beat them like a left-handed person, in reverse of what's normal, so I lost the job right after that. They said if the eggs get beaten in the wrong direction the cake won't rise.

Mama doesn't mind that Amelia and I are friends. I always heard that if you are walking in the street and see a black person you should throw them a kiss and that day you can wish for anything and it will come true, because black people bring good luck. I don't believe in that; to me they are black people, not lucky charms.

For a few months now, Mama has been cutting up our old bath towels and some other thick fabric she bought and making little square towels of one foot by one foot. It's a big secret. I have asked her twice what they are for and she said, "In due time, you will find out."

I was invited to Amelia's party downstairs. Amelia's family likes to wear perfume, and they are always having parties where they serve champagne with fresh fruit inside tall glasses and the music is loud and lively, people dance and everybody smiles and is friendly.

I asked Mama why we don't bathe with perfume and have parties like that, since it's so much fun.

She said that black people sweat a lot, and that's why they have to use perfume; we don't have that problem to worry about. And their music is always too loud because they are loud people and have no responsibilities.

I don't agree. But I didn't say anything. I am afraid she will stop me from visiting them.

Amelia tells me everything; her mom and sisters all work, they all have regular jobs, it's only on weekends that they like to be happy and celebrate life with their friends. Amelia also confided in me about the boy that lives on the second floor of our building. One of her sisters and her were invited to a small gathering at their apartment upstairs and Claudio the white boy, as she called him, took her into his bedroom and they kissed each other on the lips. She confides in me, we tell each other everything. We have become sisters. We made a little pinhole on each other's finger and we held them together so that our blood could run from one into the other. We are blood sisters and friends forever.

Down the street from Grandma's house there is a bakery that sells fun candy. They are very expensive, probably because they have liquor inside. These candies must be made for children, because they are very cute in the form of a little baby wrapped in a blanket. They are made of hard sugar and come in pink, blue, yellow or green. I always buy two of them, a boy and a girl. It was a great surprise when I bit into one for the first time and delicious sweet liquor came out. I can only buy them once in a blue moon because I also love potato chips and chocolates. Chocolates are my very favorite and also a lot of fun to buy. They are sold at the cigarette and magazine shops where they offer the chocolate game board, which is a large punchboard and the way it works is you push with a pin one of the many dots on the punchboard and on the other side it tells you which chocolate bar you get. I hope someday I will get the grand prize, which is a box of chocolates. Most of the time I get small or medium size chocolate bars, and once in awhile, very rarely I get the super-size chocolate bar. It's all luck.

Aunt Heydee is a very independent person, but when it comes to the arts she is soft like butter. She is very sensitive. Two weeks ago she came home crying as she described a young boy singing opera on a street corner. He didn't sing like everybody else, according to Aunt Heydee, he sang like Caruso. Then she reconsidered her words, "No, he sang like an angel. I have to do something to help him; he needs someone to look out for his interests. He will never make it alone. He will be lost in this city. I can't allow that to happen; it would be a crime!" And she left to go looking for him, hoping to find him so she could take care of him or even adopt him if necessary. She came back a few hours later crying. This time she was hysterical, because she couldn't find him anywhere.

She has been looking for the young singer daily, asking people in the street if they had seen him. Everybody has forgotten the little boy with the golden voice and he is nowhere to be found. Most likely he went back to his hometown and back to sowing the fields, disillusioned and heartbroken. There is no future in a big city like Lisbon, even if he sang better than Caruso.

I don't like beer. Mama says beer will put some meat on my bones and best of all it will make me less constipated. I tried and tried to drink it, but it makes me throw up every time. Finally she gave up making me drink beer with my meals because I throw up the meal with the beer. Beer is gross and wine makes me sick. Liquor is the only thing I like, and my favorite is still anise.

Mama has a hard time finding a good maid. She tries to pick someone nice when they answer the newspaper ad, but she always gets the wrong person. One after another, either they have syphilis, are pregnant, or steal everything they can while we are sleeping. Sometimes they get fired because they can't cook or they don't present the food in an appetizing manner. Mama is very picky about presentation; she says food should appeal first by the way it looks and smells, and burning it is not acceptable. I was sorry when Teresa left us to go back home, but her family needed her. Once in a while we get one that decides that she is going to flirt with Papa by using very sexy smiles, or wearing low-cut blouses displaying the breasts, brushing against him while serving dinner at the table, or saying naughty things like, "Mr. Wartenberg, would you like some more of my delicious noodles with your fish?"

Mama catches on very quickly when that happens. Matter of a fact, she no longer hires anyone that is young or good-looking, they have to be over fifty years old, and if they have a mustache that's a good requisite to getting hired. I notice things like that.

Over the years Mama has become a professional expert in hiring and firing maids. For example, if they wear black stockings, she makes them take the stockings off and she looks at their legs for syphilis sores. We had one that was sent to Uncle Augusto because her belly was getting bigger everyday. She told Mama that was the result of eating too many fava beans. Mama's suspicions were correct and the new maid was fired. Then there was the one that would not take the garbage out by five in the morning. Mama told her that if she didn't take the garbage out she could not work for us anymore. That night Mama woke up hearing the maid opening the back door about five in the morning, and she told Papa, "Well, it sounds like Josefina is taking the garbage out like she is supposed to do."

When we got up in the morning Josefina had not only taken the garbage out, but she had also broken into Mama's linen closet and taken all the bed sheets and blankets and some other things that Mama had under lock and key. Mama cried a lot over that, but later in the evening she brought up to us her favorite proverb, "It's okay to lose the rings as long as we don't lose the fingers."

Mama still gets emotional over stuff that happens but then quickly she turns it around to the positive side, which is good otherwise she would go crazy.

It was so scary when I heard Mama screaming the other night as she ran down the hallway and into the dining room next to the bathroom. She was crying as she grabbed Papa. "I just saw my father in the pantry room, just standing there." Papa hugged her and tried to calm her down, then she went and had some more calming medicine that she gets from Uncle Augusto to help her with her nerves.

I didn't say anything but I believe that Mama has hallucinations. Every time she says something hurts, the doctors don't believe her; they tell her it's all nerves. They have her on all kinds of pills so she doesn't complain. I hate pills, needles, and doctors, but not Uncle Augusto.

I am looking forward to the summer so that I can go to the Feira Popular, a very famous Amusement Park. Every year we spend at least one afternoon there. We never have enough money with us for rides or to buy cotton candy or even a clay toy, but I enjoy seeing the other people screaming as they ride down the roller coaster, and most of all I can spend hours watching the motorcycle man going around and around inside his cage without falling off his bike. That proves that gravity exists. If Mama goes to the Feira Popular it's usually at night with Papa. But once in a while she will go with my brothers and me. She will buy us cotton candy, which I really like a lot, and I am allowed one ride. My favorite is the merry-go-round.

I love the smell of cotton candy, hotdogs and the clay pottery brought in from the countryside. Pottery has a certain smell that I love; I don't know how to explain it.

Max-Leão and I are attending a home-study group, at the house of a retired teacher that is very close to where

Grandma Rica used to live. Mama is worried that if I don't brush up on geometry, math, and French and Portuguese grammar I am going to forget everything by the time I get to go to High School. The classes at the home-study group are like a refresher course. Max-Leão comes with me because he is not a good student in high school and he can use all the tutoring he can get. It takes us about 45 minutes to walk there from our house, but I like it because I get to chat with Max- Leão. They teach us math, drawing, geometry, history, French, and Portuguese grammar.

Our teacher Julia is an assistant to the old teacher, and she is in charge of three other kids besides my brother and me. She is a young girl with lots of facial acne and wears dresses that are very low cut and tight, which makes her breasts stick out just like the beautiful German actress Romy Schneider, her favorite actress. Julia is very romantic and loves romantic movies. During our two-hour lunch break, I look forward to sitting next to her as she describes with the flair of a storyteller, the whole movie she saw over the weekend, starring Romy Schneider. It's better than going to the movies; sometimes it takes more than a week for her to finish the story because she describes every scene with perfect accuracy paying special attention to all the details, no matter how small they might be, and if any of us likes a particular part, and wants to hear it again, she is more than happy to repeat it.

Max-Leão and I were walking back to our house from the home-study group, we were talking about the power of the mind, and he said he wondered if that is possible.

"Of course it is possible; I do it every day. I can make anything happen!" I said that, bragging about something that I knew nothing about. I just wanted to impress him.

"You can't do that," he said, "you are lying!"

"Okay," I said to him, as we were just crossing in front of a school where kids were running down the steps, "Do you see that kid in the white uniform, watch him. He is going to fall down the steps," and I pointed my finger at the boy. The boy tripped half way down the steps and fell.

We didn't stop. We kept walking rapidly and Max-Leão became very quiet and so did I. Max-Leão was impressed, but I knew that I had lied. I could not possibly have guessed the boy was going to fall; it simply happened that he tripped at the moment I pointed at him; it was just luck of the draw.

Summer of 1957

I am supposed to believe that Max-Leão writes short stories and poetry about life. He is twelve years old, hates to write, and has had no life experience of any kind. I know that he is not writing this stuff. It has to be a ghost that has possessed him since he knows as much as I do about sex. That means he knows nothing. Supposedly he wrote *"Women - women are born to be an instrument of possession, like the flowers being sold, like the long and time-consuming kisses, like the rose that upon being held is soft but frail; petals fall to my feet."* Give me a break!

This was a real strange day for me. I went to the bathroom this morning and blood was coming out of my vagina for no reason. I debated for a while as to what to do and finally gave up and called Mama. I felt so ashamed having to tell her that I was bleeding from there of all places.

She was not surprised and said, "Finally I can give you my present." And she left running down the hallway.

A few minutes later she came back running with a huge paper package tied up with a rope. I thought, *what a weird time to give me a present, as I am dying.* I opened the package puzzled. It was one dozen square cotton towels, the ones she had been sewing for some time. How in the world did she know that this was going to happen to me? I was very impressed by her intuition. Then she told me that all young girls start bleeding at twelve or thirteen years old, it's called menstruating and that is how they become women. It's absolutely normal to bleed every month for about five or six days. Now I really have to be careful, she told me. If a boy comes up to me and kisses me, I will become pregnant and a baby will grow inside my belly. Her advice was for me to stay away from boys and wait until I am married to get pregnant. Then she showed me how to fold the napkin and pin it to my underwear with two safety pins, one in the back and another in the front.

She took me into the sunroom and handed me a brand-new big metal bucket, saying, "From now on, this is your own personal bucket. You put cold water inside and your napkins get to soak in the water for a few hours, then you take the napkins out and rinse them again in the bucket till the blood is all gone."

This is so disgusting; being a girl is really the pits. I wish I were a boy instead.

When I was younger, a friend from school told me that her brother's penis would expel white-like fluid every so often. She knew about these things because her mother used to get upset and yell at her brother when she would make his bed and find the sheets all sticky. As far as I know my brothers don't have that problem, because not every boy has that happening to him. I think that if I had a choice, I would rather have a discharge of white sticky stuff once in a blue moon than a bloody mess every month for the rest of my life.

Last week, Mama gave Rosa our maid some money to spend with us at the Feira Popular; it was enough for one ride for each of us. I picked the twirling ride, it goes around and around and you get sucked up on your back into the railing due to the force of gravity I believed it was going to be a pleasant ride. I didn't like it at all; it made me dizzy and sick to my stomach. They had to stop the machine and let everybody next to me out, because I threw up and the wind blew the vomit around. They screamed at me and everybody was angry, but it was the guy's fault for not stopping the motor when I started to yell, "Please stop! Please stop, I am going to throw up!" Nope, they didn't believe me.

We have gone back to Eiriceira. It was a unanimous vote, as we all like this little fishing village a lot more than Costa da Caparica, even if it is for only one month this summer. I will never see João again. I believe it's better this way. After all, I must sacrifice myself, because this is true love, like Don Pedro and the Spanish princess Donna Inez: They both lived hidden in a villa in Coimbra, because his father, the King of Portugal, did not approve of Don Pedro's choice. There was a possibility that someday she could become the queen of Portugal when Don Pedro took over the throne, and that could never be allowed to happen. So his father the king paid two criminals to kill Donna Inez while Don Pedro was away from the villa. They killed her right in front of her children. She cried out for mercy, but they had been paid good money for killing her. Don Pedro went crazy when he learned about what happened to his beloved, the mother of his children. He hunted down the two men and proceeded to kill them personally by ripping the heart out of one through the front of his chest and the other one through his back. Later on, when Don Pedro became the king, he had the body of Donna Inez taken out from the grave and seated on the throne and everyone paid homage and kissed the hand of his dead beloved. Then he made special arrangements for Donna Inez to be buried again. He buried her making sure that her tomb would face his when he was buried so that when they returned again at the end of the world, the first thing they would see would be each other.

It's too bad he stayed crazy and wasted his life drinking and hanging around with the people of the streets never to do anything else with his life, except drinking, suffering, and crying. The villa where Donna Inez was murdered became known as "A Quinta das Lágrimas," the Villa of Tears.

All the friends I had here in Eiriceira have not returned this summer; even Madalena will be leaving in two weeks. I heard her father telling Mama and Aunt Heydee, who was visiting us, that he knew Madalena was a virgin because when she pisses it comes out delicately, not hard and loud. If she ever lost her virginity, he would immediately know from the sound of her peeing that she was no longer a virgin.

I am glad that he never heard me, because my peeing can be soft, and sometimes if I'm holding on for a long time it is loud and I am a virgin like Aunt Heydee, who has never been married.

Aunt Heydee came by to visit us for two days, and as always something wonderful happens when she is around. She took my two brothers and me for a country hike! I had never been to a hike.

We went up the road and into some farmland and then she pointed to the field, "Look, corn to take home!"

We looked at her surprised since it was not ours to take.

"Yeah, behind a fence!" said my brother José.

"Yeah," she said, "except these two corns are sticking out of the fence." And she pulled them out. We all ran down the hill laughing and when we got home she boiled the corn and it was split into six pieces among all of us. I love corn!

Papa visits us on weekends; he gets here late Friday and leaves Sunday evening. Mama and Papa invited me to go to the movies with them. The last time I remember going to the movies together was a long time ago, to see "Snow White," for my birthday. But this weekend, what I thought was going to be great turned out really dumb. It was an American movie, starring the blonde American actress Lana Turner. About halfway through the movie the actors, young teenagers, were having a party when the parents were not home. They were drinking and some were kissing and dancing in very close embrace and I thought, *wow, my parents are really getting cool.*

Then Papa said to Mama, in his very German accent, "This is no good for our young daughter. They are going to start fornicating in this scene, let's leave right now."

Mama agreed.

How could they do this to me, in the middle of a great American movie? Here I was, thinking they were taking me out like a grownup, and instead I was being treated like a child. So what, they were kissing each other, big deal. Now I will never know the end of the movie. When are they going to treat me like an adult, like a human being, with rights? One of our beach neighbors came by this morning holding in her arms her granddaughter who is only three years old. She told us that the little girl has anemia, and she is going to die very soon, maybe in a month or two. I stared at the child who was smiling at everybody. I don't understand why God allows her to be born and die so soon. I guess that nothing lasts forever, not even a little girl for her grandmother's sake. I'm not going to let this bother me. I can't help her. I don't care anymore.

I spend most of my time sitting on the sand and staring at the ocean. I like watching the waves and the way they hit the rocks, intertwining under them with such force that they shoot straight up into the air, each wave trying to out-do the previous one.

I like to dream, and see the sunsets. I am awake to everyone that goes by because my eyes are open, and they see my body sitting on the rocks or below on the soft sand, but I'm not there in spirit, only physically. I'm getting so good at it that I can do it even when there are people around me. It feels good to be by myself. I don't need anyone or anything, I am not happy and I am not sad, I am here and I am not, just like the little girl that is going to die very soon.

That was some incredible storm last night. I woke up hearing the sound of wind and ocean hitting the rocks and moving them below us. It was louder and deeper than thunder. It felt like the earth was moving, and since our house is right on the tip of the cliff I woke up wondering if we were still on the cliff or floating on the ocean. We went to look outside our front door and the beach was gone. The noise we had heard during the night was from a huge storm that came and took all the sand off the beach and brought in huge rocks. There wasn't a grain of sand to be found, it had all been swept clean. There were only rocks, rocks of all sizes.

The owner of the beach was sitting on the ground crying. He had lost his livelihood because he cannot collect rent for the cloth cabanas when there's no sand to stick them into. There is no beach to speak of anymore.

Everyone felt very sorry for him. Mama and the other women promised him that we would stay until the end of the month and still pay for the cabanas, even though it was very uncomfortable for us to sit on stones.

The good side to all of this was the enormous world of sea creatures that appeared before our eyes. Lots and lots of seafood to be cooked daily and the most beautiful seashells we have ever seen were found between the rocks. Mama is going to use them to sew as decoration for my clothing and to make necklaces for everyone. Max-Leão, José and I get to pick up a lot of crustaceous sea creatures. We put them into our beach pails and take them home to be boiled in salty water. At night, my brothers and I sit outside the house on its steps and with a pin we pull the tender morsels out of the shells, eating the delicious bits of the ocean. I love the taste and fresh smell of the sea.

Good news! A German company has hired Papa as their representative in Portugal. Now we can start paying back all the money that Aunt Heydee, Encarnação, and Uncle Augusto loaned us through the years. Papa will have his own office, and Mama will be helping him at work when we get back to Lisbon. She told us that Papa was chosen from among hundreds of other men because of his honesty and high morals. The company sponsors Portuguese and foreign artists that paint with their mouth or feet because they have no hands or arms. The German company uses the handicapped artist's work for postcards and calendars, and uses the money they receive to help these artists and their families with income. Everybody benefits from it; the artists, our family, and many Portuguese employees that will have steady work and benefits. Most important, Papa will be getting paid every month a regular salary.

Mama already made all the arrangements for when we get back to Lisbon. The plans are set for a bathtub, a full-time maid once again, and I will be going to a private all-girls high school. I will be starting this October. It is expensive, but necessary if I am to stay untouched by *goims* until I marry cousin Alberto from North America. The high school is right across Encarnação's house, a few blocks from where we live. This will be very handy on cold winter days when I have to walk back and forth in the rain.

I am very happy that soon I will be in a real school. I will be using a white uniform, which is very good, since my clothing is very meager. Mama also likes the idea of a uniform; I won't need a wardrobe to go to school. I only need a pair of decent shoes.

Since our sandy beach has washed away into the ocean, I have been walking more often to the tourist beach, which is just past the beach used by the fishermen. Nobody uses it because you might step on a fishing hook or a dead fish, and we all know that this beach belongs only to the fishermen arriving with their fresh catch very early in the morning. There is no pier, they leave their colorful fishing boats of all sizes against the back wall where the tide is not suppose to reach and they leave their nets drying all over the sand, and through the day you are guaranteed to see a few old fishermen in their typical fishing gear sewing their nets by their boats, pulled along the seashore.

It's very hard for me to get up super early in the morning just to see the fishing boats coming into the bay. I did it once with Max-Leão and they gave us a couple of sardines for helping them to pull the nets ashore. I don't like sardines; they are too fat and, as always, oily or greasy stuff makes me nauseous.

Mama loves sardines and so do her sisters. She told us about the time when she was with her sister Heydee spending the summer at the beach. Like us they had helped some fishermen to pull the fishing nets. A couple of handsome fishermen not only gave them some sardines afterwards, but they also prepared a small fire, where they broiled the fish right there on the sand.

Mama and Aunt Heydee were young and very beautiful and every man that saw them would fall madly in love with them; the fishermen were no exception. Two handsome fishermen sat next to them on the sand talking to them, and Aunt Heydee became so absorbed in the conversation that she didn't notice that Mama was eating the sardines, chewing the fish heads, sucking up all the juices, then she would throw what was left of the fish into the bucket right next to her, which had some water in it. As the sardines were being put into the bucket of water, their heads would swell again, and Aunt Heydee — who only had goo-goo eyes for one of the handsome fishermen — wasn't paying attention to which bucket she was taking her sardines from. She was taking the sardines from the wrong bucket, chewing on the same fish head that Mama had just spat out. As much as I love chewing on fish heads myself, I have to admit this story is the grossest I ever heard.

There is only one story that's even more disgusting than the sardine story. This is actually not a story, it is a famous Portuguese joke based on a true fact that in order to go to medical school you are either rich or starving to death since you can't afford to pay for food after you pay the tuition. Also, it could never be a true story since it is just too disgusting to be true and I only laughed the first time I heard it. Max-Leão told me about it. Two very poor medical students attending the University of Coimbra in the north of Portugal were dissecting a human body at the lab. When they opened the dead man's stomach they found it to be full of rice. The dead man's last meal had obviously been rice, and it was still warm, the sight of warm rice made the two hungry medical student's mouths water.

Manuel said to Mário the other student, "There's a phone call for you out in the hallway, you better go and get it."

While Manuel was out, Mário used his hands to dig the rice out of the dead man's open stomach. Suddenly Manuel came back and realized he had been tricked as he saw Mário with a mouth full of rice. Exasperated because he wanted the rice for himself, he said to Mário, "How disgusting! How utterly disgusting! Eating the rice from a dead man's stomach! It makes me want to puke."

Mário realized that Manuel was right and got sick to his stomach and started to throw up back into the dead man's stomach, and then he walked away to clean himself.

Manuel had done well at tricking his friend out of the room and with a big smile he began eating the puked rice from the cadaver's stomach.

When we got back to Lisbon, Mama sent Papa with me to buy me shoes and a raincoat for when school starts. Now, that was some trip to downtown Lisbon. He took me to the best store, the one where tourists buy their stuff. A lady came up to us and he said, "My daughter needs a raincoat for the winter. Show me the best one you have in this store."

She did. She guaranteed that not a drop of water will go through this type of gabardine material and it will last forever. It is double-faced; one side is light gray, mostly for winter use, the other side is a soft cool blue, more for the spring look as was my fancy that day. It fits perfect. And it has a belt to match both sides. Finally I can show my waist. Everything else I have to wear is big and wide, to last years and years of use. The shoes are made of real leather and they don't really fit comfortably on my big feet, but the lady said that they would stretch the more I use them.

Papa was happy with his purchases and so was I. When Mama saw the bill with the amount he had paid, she almost fainted. She said she would never; ever again send me out with Papa to buy anything, because he had just blown a small fortune. If she had known he was a spendthrift, she would have taken me instead.

Thank God she didn't. I love the raincoat. And the shoes, according to the shoe sales lady, won't hurt my feet once they are broken in.

We are so modern! We have a brand new bathtub and a heating system above it which, upon lighting it with a match, heats up the water to take the bath with. Papa was very patient at showing us how to use it. Papa also bought a washing machine! The fun starts when the clothes go through the wringer to take the water off and they come out almost dry. No more twisting by hand.

The maid called it sissy stuff, as she would rather wash everything by hand the old-fashioned way.

If technology keeps going like this, who knows what the future will bring, another ten years and we will be visiting other planets. I want to travel in space so badly!

Autumn of 1957

I am so glad I was not born a princess. I know that miracles can happen and sometimes a person can become a queen or a princess by marrying someone from royalty. I hope that will never happen to me. What's the use of being rich when you have to constantly watch what you do and say in public and every move you make has to be dignified? I saw poor Elizabeth II of England when she was visiting our country this year, and she looked like a stuffed doll smiling and waving her hand back and forth as she peeked out of the old coach during the royal parade down the Avenida da Liberdade. I can only imagine how smelly and hot it must be inside an old coach built in 1820. The poor thing; she would have been better off walking.

I have been to the Coach Museum several times, and I always leave with a headache from the impregnated musty mold of the antique coaches. Even though, I have to admit that I like seeing them and playing in my mind the ways of yesterday, when without a horse you couldn't travel too far.

Some of these coaches were enormous, like monsters, and after one trip they were done for.

I have read many books concerning the lives of the aristocratic and it's not a pretty picture. I would never want to be a princess because I would have to follow the laws and rules of behavior as dictated by the royal people and their ancestors.

Mama vomits a lot. Trying to lose weight is not easy for her. She eats her meal, followed by, "I'll be right back." And she runs to the bathroom and vomits all the food she ate. I can hear her vomiting into the toilet, it sounds horrible. It must hurt her throat every time she does that. I don't like to vomit. She bought some Italian sticks made of hard dried bread and she has been eating them instead of real bread, but it doesn't seem to help her to lose weight. It's horrible to see her suffer like that on account of food. I wish I could help, but I don't know how. It makes me sad when I don't have a solution to a problem.

I started the all-girl's private high school across from Encarnação's house. This is really the best school I could ever imagine. I am so happy with the school, my raincoat, and the new shoes. There are about five to six girls per class and the teachers know each of us by name! There's a teacher for each subject, and each teacher loves to teach her subject. I am even enjoying science. There's a lab for science experiments, there's sewing, gymnastics, and ballet classes. Portuguese, Latin, French, and English are the languages. I don't care for French but I love English. I can't escape taking Algebra, Geometry, and Geography, but World History makes up for all the subjects that I don't like. I have counted by my fingers twelve different subjects at school, and I love every one of them, even if I still have lots of difficulty with Math and Algebra. Anything with numbers is a nightmare.

The classrooms are so small that no matter where I sit, I can hear and see a lot better. The girls are very grown up, and most of them have boyfriends and they go to parties at each other's homes and they have their own little cliques to which I don't belong because I am different. I have no boyfriend, no parties at my house, no friends, and no freedom of any kind. Even though we all wear the same uniforms they can tell that, underneath I don't have pretty clothes bought from fancy stores like they do. My clothes are made at home. I wear my hair straight because when I use hair curlers I get a headache. I don't go to the beauty parlor because Mama can't afford to pay for it, and besides, every time I get my hair curled, they burn my hair, my scalp, and the top of my ears with the chemical they use for making the hair curl. The beauticians say I have delicate hair and I am allergic to the chemicals touching my skin. At school they call me "existentialist" because I am different from my schoolmates. Even though I was born in Portugal my last name makes me a foreigner.

I walked home repeating in my head over and over again the joke I heard in school today. My friend Beatriz is the one that told me and I thought it was really funny. I waited until everybody was seated for dinner so that I would have a nice-sized audience. My intent was to impress Mama and Papa with my humor, since a few years ago Papa was very impressed with my tongue clicking at the roof of my mouth. Both of them were amazed at my creativity and had laughed heartily. I wanted to make them laugh again.

We were all about to start eating the vegetable bean soup when I said, "There was this young girl sitting on top of a tree and she wasn't wearing underwear because she was very poor and couldn't afford to buy it. A man walked under the tree and looked up and felt sorry for the young girl and said to her, 'Here pretty girl, take this 25 *centavos* and buy yourself some underwear.' She ran home happily to tell her mother what happened. The next day the mother figured that would be an easy way to make a living so she got herself on top of the tree without underwear and waited patiently for the same kind gentleman to walk by under the tree. That day it happened he was walking by and happened to look up at the tree and when he saw she was not wearing underwear he said to her, 'You poor woman, take this 50 *centavos* and go get yourself a shave.'"

I barely made it to the punch line trying to control my laughter.

Papa didn't laugh; he got very angry. "This is a very offensive joke to tell your parents."

Mama seemed to have a smile on her face, but added, "You shouldn't tell jokes like these at the table. It's in very poor taste."

Papa stopped eating and continued to lecture. "An educated and proper-mannered girl would never talk like that. Verónica, you have disappointed me."

My tears fell in the soup and I swore to myself that I would never tell a joke or open myself to them. This is a lesson to learn, they are my fuddy-duddy parents, not my friends.

According to Mama, calf brains are guaranteed to help increase intelligence and clear the thought process during school exams. I don't know if that actually makes me smarter, but Mama says eating them is good for my brains. I personally don't believe it, but I like their taste when they get stewed in wine sauce. The other thing that makes me laugh — and I only take it to make Mama happy — is the medicine that she gives me in a tablespoon before I leave the house to take the tests in school. I entered the kitchen one day and I saw her preparing the concoction, sugar and water! I know I am not smart, but I'm not that stupid either. She says it's a calming medicine from Uncle Augusto's medicine cabinet. She doesn't know that I saw her making it; Mama likes to use psychology but it doesn't work with me, she lies.

"Ah, Burt Lancaster, now that's a man that takes my breath away," said Mama as she delicately sipped the tea from her china cup. Aunt Heydee and Aunt Simy were visiting us. They were all having tea and butter cookies.

"Oh, no," said Aunt Simy, "For me there's no one like Kirk Douglas and his cute dimpled chin."

"All American movie stars are handsome," said Aunt Heydee in all her wisdom.

Mama turned to me and asked, "I am curious, Verónica, who do you like as a man?"

"Jerry Lewis!" I responded without blinking an eye and knowing well in advance that was not the answer they wanted to hear.

"Why, in heavens?" said Aunt Simy, looking at me as if I was an odd ball.

"He is a twit, a nerd," they said almost unanimously, their faces showing complete disappointment.

I had to explain. "He makes me laugh!"

"That's not a normal man. How can a girl your age like a man that acts and looks like a clown?" said Aunt Ligia.

And then to my surprise Mama defended me. "It's okay that she likes Jerry Lewis, she is still at the age of innocence. She enjoys his humor and appreciates it. That's fine, Verónica." And she smiled at me.

My goodness, Mama sometimes is truly a wonderful person, she has moments that I could kiss her, but I didn't. I am not going to show any weakness towards her; every time I do I am sorry later on. If I stay hard on the inside she can't hurt my feelings. I am so confused.

My friend Amelia and her family went back to Africa. We cried a lot this morning as we hugged each other and said goodbye forever. I will miss them, their perfume, the gay lively attitude, the loud African music, and most of all Amelia. She will live forever in my heart.

Winter of 1958

I like storytelling, and I don't mind when one is told over and over again; but there are a few corny ones that Mama is always more than happy to tell, like the "Ten Little Friends."

There was this woman that had gotten married, and when her husband would come home from work, she had been sleeping all day and was too tired to do any housework. The poor husband would come home for lunch and she was still sleeping. He would come home for dinner and she had done nothing all day but sleep. She didn't do any housewife duties. Dinner was never ready; the house was always dirty and dusty. She was just plain lazy.

Then one day a fairy godmother appeared to her and said, "What's your wish?"

And the woman said, "I need help to take care of the house and have everything done by the time my husband gets home, the dishes cleaned, the food ready, the clothes ironed, you know, the usual housewife duties."

And the fairy godmother said, "Okay my dear, your wish is granted, I will give you ten little invisible magical friends to help you with all the chores, but you must get up early and help them, otherwise they will not help you either."

The next morning, the woman couldn't wait to get up early like the good fairy had advised her to, and she made her husband breakfast, and after he left to go to work she started dusting, and then after washing the dirty clothes in the tub and hanging them outside to dry, she put them away to be ironed in the afternoon. Then she arranged some fresh flowers on the table after preparing lunch, and she got all cleaned up for her husband who was delighted to see lunch ready.

Then he went back to work and she did the dishes and scrubbed and waxed the wooden floors and did the ironing and made a gourmet dinner after dusting the furniture and washing the windows. She noticed that by that evening she had done all her duties. The ten invisible little friends were definitely her best friends since she had everything done at the end of the day, just like she was supposed to. Thanks to her ten invisible friends, she was even dressed pretty and her hair looked really nice and she didn't smell of onions or garlic, only perfume, and when her exhausted husband got home that night she had his favorite drink ready for him.

This went on day after day, month after month, and year after year, and they had five children and they all lived happily ever after. Who were her ten friends? Who could have possibly helped this woman to become a good wife and later a good mother? One may ask? Well, I have to pause and give it some thought as if this is the very first time I heard the story. I make believe that I am thinking about the answer — that's half the fun— and then Mama lifts her hands in the air and opens her fingers wide, saying, "Her ten little fingers, of course!"

Mama took me out for a surprise. She would not tell me what it was all about. She loves mystery and she kept saying, "You will see. You will see, be patient!"

We reached the fourth floor of an old apartment house around the corner from where we live, and a very old woman dressed in black from head to toes opened the door and let us in. Her place was exactly the way I imagine a witch's house to be. I felt like I was inside a dark forest, smelly and dusty, with lots and lots of costumes and hats and everything one can imagine from days of forgotten times, the times of queens and princes and fairy tales. Nothing looked real. In the kitchen she was probably brewing magic potions, the aroma of her cooking was unrecognizable. Hanging on the walls and all over the tables and chairs and everywhere were costumes, masks, and hats in complete chaotic disarray.

The most elaborate and expensive wardrobe was hanging along the left side of the long room and it covered what was once a window. Mama told her that she was on a very tight budget and asked her to show us the least expensive outfits. It all looked good to me. I picked from the non-expensive rack a gipsy outfit. Mama agreed. The price was within her budget. It's going to be *Carnaval* in a few days, and I will have a real costume, like all the other kids. This is the real thing!

Mama had everything planned; she had matinee tickets for all of us. My make-up was a real workout for Mama and Aunt Heydee. It wasn't easy to make my straight hair get curly like a gipsy would wear around her face. Red lipstick, green eye shadow, black eyelash coloring, and of course the most important part of all of the make-up, the *piece de resistance*, a black mole on my right cheek was drawn carefully with Mama's personal black pencil she uses for drawing her own mole when she goes somewhere special with Papa. When they finally were finished with me, Mama took a deep breath of contentment, "So this is the way Verónica will look like when she gets to be an adult. Not bad with make-up."

I think that Mama enjoyed seeing me look pretty.

We all had fun costumes, Max-Leão was a pirate with an eye patch and José a cowboy, Aunt Heydee made her own dress out of something, nobody knows what or how, but she looked like a queen. Even though *Carnaval* is meant to be for kids only, there's no law that says that adults can't have fun. In Brazil, adults get all dressed up and celebrate *Carnaval* with a huge parade. Mama didn't want to go with us. She only had five tickets and she sent the maid with us instead, to watch us. The show was an American musical and it showed the way Americans live, always singing and dancing every time they go out to a restaurant or out into the field to work on the farm.

Intermission was horrible. The kids and the adults with them were throwing little bags full of hard corn tied to an elastic string so that they could hit you in the head with it and immediately retrieve it before you could catch them. Each hit was very painful. The bags of corn felt more like stones. I didn't have corn bags to fight back so I was at their mercy. If that's entertainment, they must be mad. It wasn't a laughing matter. I could feel the lumps on my skull starting to form. I promised myself that I would never again go to one of these *Carnaval* events with other kids. I'm too grown up for that. No wonder, Mama didn't join us, she is smarter than I give her credit for.

Aunt Heydee agreed with me that getting hit over the head over and over again with a bag of dried corn was a cruel and childish way to enjoy the *Carnaval*. She took my

Getting Hit with Dried Corn.

picture outside the theatre and told me I looked too beautiful to go home. She sent my brothers home with the maid, and took me to her favorite dance hall so that I could show off my outfit. She said I could go with her but I was not allowed to dance, and because of my age I would not be allowed to enter the dancehall. She got me to sit on a fainting couch outside the main ballroom and from there I was able to watch her dance. Aunt Heydee can dance to any tune, she has a natural beat.

I sat there thinking about Mama when she was young and used to come to places like this with her sisters. She has told us several times about the young man that came up to her and said, "Would you like something to drink?"

And she said, "Whiskey!"

He came back with a whiskey and then asked her to dance with him and she said, "No, I do not want to dance with you!"

And when he asked her why not, she responded by saying, "Because you are not my type, and I despise you."

I don't like that story. It bothers me that she brags about this event and she is even proud of being arrogant and harsh as a young woman. I hope I never become like her.

I decided not to think about things like that, and watch all those grown-ups twirling under the shiny crystal chandeliers and white stone pillars which reminded me of an old Greek palace. A man came up to me and asked me to go inside with him to dance.

Feeling my cheeks getting red with embarrassment I told him, "I am sorry but I'm not allowed to do that, I'm only here because I am waiting for my Aunt Heydee, who is dancing over there." And I pointed to her.

He said he was going to be right back.

Not ten minutes passed by and Aunt Heydee came up to me and grabbed my hand. "C'mon, let's get out of here," she said hurriedly. "If your mother finds out that I brought you to this place, she will have my head."

I started to tell Aunt Heydee about the man that had approached me and she cut me off saying, "Yeah, I know all about him, he is a lawyer. And he had the balls to tell me that he had a lot of money and would pay anything to dance with you. I told him that you are only thirteen years old, and not for sale."

I have stopped eating chocolates and potato chips since the beginning of the year. I get 30 *escudos* per month as my allowance. I don't go to the movies, because if I go twice in one month I don't have anymore money, and my goal now is to save enough money to buy a birthday gift for Papa in April and hopefully for Mama next December. I am on a mission. I have my eye on a small diamond pin for Papa's tie and a colorful real stone broach for Mama; this is going to impress them both. I know they love me but when they get these presents they will love me even more. I get a regular paycheck from working weekends and evenings at Papa's office. I work all the weekends; the more hours, the more money I can put together. I need a lot of money if I want to buy the gifts. I address and stuff envelopes with postcards and calendars and information on the artists. People are amazed at how these artists paint beautiful artwork using the brush with their mouth or feet. They were born without arms and some lost their limbs in a car accident and have become wheelchair-bound, without any other means to make a living. Papa and the German company make a living from giving these people a second chance. Life can be brutal unless we make the best we can with what God gives us daily.

For the last three months I spent most of my morning weekends at Cousin Marcus library. He is a distant cousin of the Ezaguy family. Probably the reason I had never heard of him or his wife until Aunt Heydee arranged for me to come to their home and use their private library.

It was my intention to read all their books until last week, when their two sons and daughter came home before I left. I felt out of place in the way I was meagerly dressed and I was also afraid to say something stupid. I tried to leave but they insisted that I stay and have lunch with them. Their maid brought us hot milk and toast and cheese. They were as nice as they could be towards me, but I knew that I didn't belong as I made every effort to eat my sandwich and not drop any crumbs on the white tablecloth. Then Michael the youngest boy said something really funny as I was drinking my milk. I couldn't help laughing along with them, except that the unexpected happened, the milk came pouring out of my nose. Everybody was laughing at me and I tried to laugh too as I was crying on the inside for being such a jerk.

Aunt Heydee told me that they were asking about me and wondering why I had stopped going to their home. I told Aunt Heydee that I finished reading all their books.

Spring of 1958

I don't like Portuguese music. The *fado* music is sad and depressing. The Portuguese are never happy when they sing, it's always the same old story, someone they love either died or is cheating on them. I'd rather listen to rock and roll. I love Elvis Presley, Big Joe Turner, Chuck Berry, Bill Haley, Paul Anka and so many I can't even count with my fingers, they are all great. They make me move and I feel happy from my toes to my head. When I hear their music on the radio, I can't sit still.

The two most painful events in my life are menstruation cramps once a month, and my birthday celebration. In my family, everything is always a big secret. Everybody most likely knows what's going on, but it's still kept a secret. So Aunt Heydee takes me to a movie matinee, that's her present for my birthday, but I'm not supposed to tell anyone because she wants everyone to think that she is on a very fixed income, which *everybody* already knows.

Then Mama comes to me and whispers, "I'm going to take you to the midday movie matinee, but I don't want you to tell anyone, and most of all not your father because he is going to take us both tonight to the movies for your birthday!"

Three times in one day I sit on a chair for a total of almost six hours, and that's when my tailbone hurts. Since I fell on my back in Eiriceira, sitting for too long is very painful to my tailbone. I am keeping my fingers crossed that when I turn fifteen years old there will be a surprise party for me with balloons and a birthday cake covered with fifteen candles, and Mama will give me a beautiful dress like Encarnação's daughters wear with a wide skirt and high heeled shoes, and in the evening I will be allowed to go dancing and I will meet a handsome young man and we will fall in love and we will get married and live happily ever after.

I was going for a walk to downtown Lisbon and had just turned at the corner of our street to go down to the Praça do Chile to take the trolley when I was inundated with a glow of sunshine, and the air become like a transparent gown that covered me with life from inside my soul to my skin and hair. I know that scientifically speaking there's no explanation, but it was like being lifted by angels and I knew that God was once again very visible to me, as life itself. Wow! What a feeling. It lasted just a few minutes but I was smiling the rest of the day. Too bad this feeling doesn't happen more often. I love it. Love it!

Mama came home very excited and told us that she had visited a fortune teller and was told that her three children would be like stars, each going in a different direction.

I don't understand why that was such good news, unless she is happy that my brothers and I are leaving home. What I wonder is where are we going? The gipsy didn't say. I don't believe they can tell the future by looking at one's hand. It all sounds to me like psychology talk. They always say the same stuff, "You have someone special in your life, you have lost someone special in your life, watch out for someone that envies you, they will try to hurt you, you will be going on a long trip — soon."

This gipsy reading was different from the usual mumbo-jumbo they always say; maybe there's something true about it and my brothers and I will be going in different directions. I hope not too far from home.

Mama made me take José to the hospital for his asthma treatment, which consists of sitting in an airtight closed box with other asthmatic people, and then they pressurize the compartment as if we were flying up in an airplane. This is supposed to help José breathe. I cried with the pressure in my ears, it hurt like hell. Mama was very nice about it when I told her. I don't have to do it again, but I have to take José for breathing treatments of some smelly stuff that's supposed to help his lungs. I am not his mother; Mama should be the one going with José not me. The smell makes me nauseous and I want to throw up every time I go with him.

Mama started sending the maid with José for the breathing treatments at the hospital, thank God for that. I don't know how José or the maid can stand that smell.

If I am going to enter the second year of high school, I will have to pass an entrance exam on all the subjects I have taken this year. This is the only way to graduate from one year to another. It is a very demanding experience. The oral and written exams are given at another school, so there's no funny business with our own teachers giving us a good grade and passing us. I have been doing slightly below average, and for me that's maximum because I am not as smart as Max-Leão or José. I don't even come close to Max-Leão's photographic memory or José's genius with math, physics and geometry. I'm barely passing everything by the seat of my pants, and that's because the teachers are very good and the classes are small and intimate. If it weren't for every single one of them being such good teachers, I would know absolutely nothing, just like when I was in primary school. The four years that I attended it was a waste of time. I never had any idea of what was really being taught and I never got a good foundation. Wearing glasses now helps me to see what's written on the blackboard, but I consider myself to be a terrible student and taking tests is pure torture. It's pathetic that during the oral exam your family can come into the school and watch you make a fool of yourself. I made Mama and Aunt Heydee promise they would sit quietly in the last row of the examining room.

For dinner last night, Mama had the maid prepare just for me calf brains stewed in wine. When we left the house this morning Mama gave me a spoonful of her usual magic potion she calls "brainpower medicine." She is a great believer in the power of suggestion, that's for sure, but I know better than that. I am going to fail the tests miserably no matter what I eat or drink. Some things are just too hard for me to do and taking tests is one of them.

Three professors sat at a long desk, and one of them called me, pronouncing my full name with difficulty. I had been watching each student get up and be questioned. They would go up to the blackboard, pick up a piece of chalk and wait until one of the examiners would give them an algebra problem. They would write down the solution to the problem, they would answer a few more questions, and wait until one of the professors said, "Thank you, you may return to your seat."

So I got up, but didn't go to the blackboard. Whatever they were going to ask me I already knew I would not have the answer, so I stood close to their desk and smiled at them, saying to myself, "What the heck am I going to do now, please dear God help me."

One of them said, "Go to the board and write down the solution to the problem I am going to give you."

I smiled again and didn't move an inch. I couldn't, since I was paralyzed with fear.

She said, "Are you hard of hearing?"

The one sitting in the middle said, "Didn't you see her name? She is a foreigner! Don't ask her to write, ask her to tell you the answer."

She did that, slowly and louder, as if that was going to make me understand her any better. With my fingers crossed behind my back I looked at them and with the most innocent look on my face I jabbered out, very sure of myself, the sounds of an instant make up language, "Oinkra, bingsy ah harling lonk zap, yahr, toom!"

The examiners asked each other, "What did she say?" All three of them were intrigued. All three of them were actually puzzled.

The examiner at the end of the table repeated the algebra question once again, looking straight at me.

I raised my hands up as if I was describing it along with my words in a manner that I hoped to come across as starting to get impatient with their ignorance of my language and I spoke this time a lot faster, "oinkrabings - yahharlinglonk-zapyahr-toom!"

"It sounds German." One of them said.

"Are you German?" Asked me the examiner on the left.

I was quick at answering, "German, yah!" I said, remembering how Papa had tried to teach my brothers and me a few simple German words one evening with no success. Frustrated, he had announced in German "Yah," and then in Portuguese he added, "my children, you sure are retarded." Then he lifted his arms in the air and left the room giving up on us.

"She looks very confident of herself and seems to know what she is saying," said one of the professors smiling at me as if he understood my dilemma.

I stood there, looking straight at them and telling myself, keep smiling and don't faint.

They talked among themselves and were convinced of my knowledge but in another language. "Thank you, miss Wartenberg, you can sit down now," they said almost in unison as they smiled at me.

I couldn't move. My feet were glued to the ground I was standing on. I questioned what they said with my eyes. The one closest to me repeated, "Sit down," and she pointed to her own chair as she got up and sat on it again.

The Algebra Test.

I went back to my seat. I got 18 out of 20 in my exam. I have never had 18 in any subject, not even history; my normal score is 11, a *passing* grade on anything I do.

I did get Mama and Aunt Heydee's full admiration for my ingenuity, and as Aunt Heydee said when we left the school, "You are truly my niece, I am Napoleão #1 but as of today, you are officially Napoleão #2."

Mama agreed. I am going places someday.

Summer of 1958

The book *I Killed my Son* by my brother Max-Leão was published. At first Aunt Heydee did not believe that it was my brother's writing, but she loves my brother so much that it didn't take Mama too long to convince her, her doubts were unjustified; after all, writing runs in our family's blood. Aunt Ligia is a writer. Cousin Augusto was a well-known writer, and there is a street in Lisbon named after him. He was very famous. Even Uncle Augusto, Mama's brother wrote poetry prior to going to medical school. He wrote the lyrics for much of Mama's original music. All the critics are in an uproar because my brother is only twelve years old but writes like a playboy. They call him a child prodigy.

I love sugar as much as I love salt. Codfish is salty but it's not my favorite food unless it's made *Gomez Sá* style, with potatoes and onions. We have codfish just about every day. Meat and chicken are only for special occasions. They say that there are at least one hundred different codfish recipes. My least favorite is boiled codfish with potatoes, carrots and cabbage, and then served sprinkled with olive oil, lemon juice, and finely chopped garlic and parsley. This has got to be the most boring food in the world. And that is Mama's favorite dish! Which means that we have to eat it too.

I like what Papa says — food is to be enjoyed for its texture and taste and presentation, and to eat like an animal without appreciating all these factors and components that go into making it special is like turning your back on a sunset.

I really like *tremoços*, a small salty yellow bean usually served free at all the taverns in Lisbon. Aunt Heydee told me that this type of legume is also called lupine bean and she believes that they were most likely introduced in Portugal when we were under the rule of the Roman Empire. Over the years I have developed a very efficient technique to eat *tremoços*. First, I put an incision on the outer skin layer with my front teeth and then I "pop" the deliciously salty seed directly into my mouth. When I was younger I would enter a tavern and grab some *tremoços*, from a small dish on the counter bar. They want their customers to keep drinking as they develop a devouring thirst for more cold beer. Lately I have been feeling too old to steal *tremoços*, so when I am in the mood for something salty and very inexpensive, I buy a small bag from a street vendor or at the grocery store. Without salt, food would have no taste.

Once upon a time there was a king who wanted to know how much his daughter truly loved him, so he asked her, and she told him, "I love you as much as salt."

He was really upset with her answer, because to him salt had no value whatsoever. Out of anger he threw her out of his kingdom — she was lucky he didn't kill her — and to prove how useless salt was, he gave her all the salt he had in storage to take with her. He didn't think that salt was important until he got his next meal. He spat out his first spoonful of soup, and when he got to the stew he realized how tasteless it was without salt. He immediately came to the realization that he needed salt or he was going to starve to death. His people were also very upset and wanted a new king, someone who had salt to share with them. Without delay, the king sent out his emissaries looking for his daughter since she had taken all the salt with her. When they found her they told her the king, her father, was very sorry and was willing to accept her back if she could only return with the salt. She did and they lived very happily ever after.

We have returned to Eiriceira for our summer vacation but we are staying at a modest house very close to the more modern beach, the one with resorts and lots of tourists; this beach has sand. The other small beach where we used to go to is still bare of any sand. Our rental house is right next to a park overlooking the ocean. The park has a roller skating rink, and swings, and steps that go down to the cliffs below us where the lobsters are kept alive for the restaurants above to use. When one walks above the rocks, it's really neat to see the lobsters underneath our feet in their manmade homes built into the rocks. The metal bars above the lobsters' cages reminds me of the Tower of Belem, the prison where political prisoners are still being put inside dungeons. Except, here the lobsters love the high tide, while the men put in the bottom of the Tower of Belem are not sea creatures and they drown. The tower just happens to be conveniently located next to the river Tejo.

My private math teacher's son was only eighteen years old when he was taken about a year ago by the government's secret police. Someone tipped them off that the boy had Communist books at home. They broke into my teacher's house and took her son away. It's been a year now and she still has no idea what happened to him. She thinks that he might have been sent to one of our African territories, like Angola or Mozambique, and put into jail. She keeps telling me, "I wonder if I will ever see him again."

I don't believe she will see him again, but I didn't tell her that. Our President Salazar is a good dictator; that's what everybody says out of fear. I am sure that my teacher's son is dead. Most likely he drowned in the Tower of Belem. Why spend for a ticket to Africa when they can kill him closer to home. Mother Nature takes care of the political prisoners, and the government officials can wash their hands; after all is it their fault that the water rises with the tide and above their cells? *Ooops! Soooooorry!*

This new beach in Eiriceira is too big for me. I don't know anyone here. I spend the days at the park sitting on one of the swings, reading. I realize that I am too shy to talk to strangers, and I'd rather read and stare at the ocean. I can stare into anything and block everything around me. I can disappear anytime I want. I just concentrate until everything around me is gone and I just float away.

I have read all the books I brought along with me from home so that the summer wouldn't be boring. Some of my favorites that I have read over and over again are; *Alice in Wonderland, David Copperfield, Oliver Twist, The Count of Monte Cristo, Arabian Nights,* and most of *The Adventures of Sherlock Holmes,* and so many more.

Someone told me there is a lady on the other side of town that rents out used books, mostly romantic novels for 10 *centavos* each. I am dying to read a romantic novel. With my allowance I will be able to read ten books this month.

I read faster than I thought. I already rented five more books. Mama gave me some change to buy ice cream. When Mama is happy she shares some of her money with me. I filled my bedroom bottom drawer with six bags of potato chips and two chocolate bars. The chocolate will not last more than a day.

I tried to roller-skate. It's not easy. I have to hold on to the railing around the skating rink, I do not want to fall. Falling on the slippery rocks a few years ago, hurt my tailbone really bad. I still can't sit for hours and hours on a hard chair without feeling pain. I can't afford to fall again, I am very careful now. Aunt Heydee is a good skater. Some kids were making fun of her and laughing because her clothing is very flamboyant and not for her age, but she started to talk to them, and by the time she was done chatting they asked her to join their group. She is an amazing person.

I was sitting on the sand this morning by our beach *cabana,* reading one of my romantic novels, when Mama appeared out of nowhere, grabbed the book out of my hand and said sternly, "Let's see what it is that you are constantly reading." Just my luck, she opened to the page where it described a passionate kiss between the two main characters. Just my luck, of all the pages she opens to, she reads that one. She called it pure trash and said now she knew why I was so uncivilized. She would not give me the book back, and prohibited me from reading anymore novels.

I was sitting on the sand acting like I was staring at the ocean, when I was actually deep into an adventure of love and danger. A handsome pirate had kidnapped me from my parents' home and he was taking me to his hidden island somewhere in Hawaii. I was debating in my mind if I really wanted to get away from him or get to know more about my future boyfriend, the pirate.

I was pulled into reality when Mama abruptly interrupted my fantasy. "I have gone through a lot of work trying to find you a friend." Then she pointed to a young woman sitting by the ocean. "Over there, her name is Clara. Go talk to her, she is looking for a friend."

I could just imagine Mama talking to a complete stranger about me, "My daughter is a nerd. She has no friends, and she is obsessed with reading trashy novels. Can you help her? Please, please!"

I got up against my will and walked over to Clara. I sat down across from her and said, "My mother wants me to talk to you."

She was twenty-three years old! She asked me if I had a boyfriend. She must be kidding! She didn't say much after that and I didn't either. Mama always passes me on to others to take care of me, like when I need to go to the dentist. Aunt Heydee is the one that goes with me. I doubt that this woman on the beach and I will ever be friends; she is old. We have nothing in common to talk about. Clara was just as uncomfortable as I was, and seemed relieved when I finally got up and said goodbye.

This afternoon I had to go to the Capital Hotel to meet with Clara, the woman from the beach. She was having lunch with other women her age. Mama told me she went through a lot of trouble to set me up for this meeting at the hotel; it was for my own good, since she wants me to stop acting like an unsocial animal. It's obvious that I will never be able to read a romantic novel again. From now on I will have to write my own love stories inside my head as I make believe that I am paying attention to the jibber-jabber around me.

When I got to the lunch meeting at the hotel, they already had finished their food and there was a small plate of ice cream that they told me to eat.

"No, thank you," I said politely.

"All kids love ice cream!" said one of them.

"I don't like ice cream," I said lying and looking straight in her eyes. How dare she call me a kid?

They kept insisting and I kept refusing and finally the ice cream melted and I felt bad that I had not eaten it, but I also felt proud I'd stuck to my guns. I am not a kid and if I choose not to eat ice cream, that's my prerogative. It's bad enough that I had to sit a whole afternoon with a bunch of older women that only talk about boyfriend experiences.

The end of this summer has been lonely and boring without books to read or anyone to talk to. My brothers are gone to do their boy stuff and I am left alone. Except for watching the sunsets while seated on the swings, I have nothing to live for.

Today a man stopped by the swing I was dangling from and said, smiling, "I see you on the swings everyday. You must really like it."

I didn't know what to say, I shook my head yes and then I ran home. I have to look for another place to hang out; he might come back, grab me and then squeeze me like a lemon. We are going back to Lisbon in one week; I am staying away from the swings from now on.

Autumn of 1958

Good news from North America! Next spring, Aunt Nelly, Mama's sister, is coming to visit us. A few months ago, her husband died from cancer. The story goes that it's been close to thirty years since she left as a young girl to marry her third Cousin Ralph, who was a pharmacist. Cousin Ralph lived in North America, New York, and he was visiting Portugal for a few days when he met Aunt Heydee at the temple in Lisbon. Aunt Heydee found out he was single and alone so she did what any kind person would do, she invited him to come home for dinner with her family that evening. It turned out that his great-grandfather was the brother of Aunt Heydee's great-grandfather, on her dad's side, which made them cousins. Two days later Cousin Ralph returned to North America. About a month later Aunt Heydee received a letter from Ralph asking for her hand in marriage. In a moment of true love and devotion to her family — who needed her more here in Portugal than abroad — she sacrificed herself by sending a letter back saying, "Thank you Cousin Ralph, but the one you must be asking the hand of in marriage has to be Nelly, since she is the most beautiful of all my sisters and also the most intelligent."

Soon Aunt Nelly got her papers in order and was waving goodbye to her family as she boarded, crying, the ship to the USA. Her mother and father were never to see her again, a small price to pay since her life was going to be easier and a lot more fruitful in North America.

Aunt Heydee cried a lot when Cousin Ralph died. He had been more than true to her over all those years, not only being a good husband to her sister Nelly, but also sending her every single month a twenty-dollar bill. Once a month she blessed his name.

In preparation for her sister's visit, Mama is having the kitchen walls painted white and the smaller front room facing the street will be Nelly's bedroom while she is staying with us. Max-Leão and José will move to the big front room with the balcony and I will be sleeping in the room next door to it where I have no privacy, because I will have two doors to be walked in at any time. Except for the bathroom door all the locks in our house don't work.

"So, Verónica, tell us about your boyfriend," Mama asked during dinner.

"What boyfriend?" She had to be kidding.

"Someone told me about him," she said winking at me. "It's very sad that you never confide in me, your own mother, and I have to find out these things from other people."

I was shocked, "I don't have a boyfriend," I said, surprised at her remarks.

"Yes you do, you have a boyfriend! Now tell us about it and stop lying about it."

My eyes started to tear as I tried very hard not to cry.

Papa came to my rescue, "Let's stop this nonsense right now. If Verónica says she has no boyfriend she doesn't have one. Verónica never lies. Daughter, I believe you!"

Wow, thank you for believing in me, you may never show any affection and for the most part I am scared of you, but sometimes you are a real dad to me, thank you. Of course I didn't say what I was thinking.

I have two girlfriends in school, Beatriz and Laura. Beatriz and I have one thing in common: we are the only two girls in school that are not Catholic. She is Protestant. We both get excused from religious class for an hour twice a week. Beatriz and I get to talk in the school's garden about our lives. She is always telling me that I am lucky to be a Jew because we were already persecuted. Now it's the Protestants turn, and someday she will wind up in a concentration camp for Protestants. I told her that since we are good friends if that happens she could hide in my house with her family.

Laura, on the other hand, became my friend because we walk home together. She has to pass my house first on the way to hers. We always leave school together and talk about the other girls who are snobs and arrive to school in their chauffeured cars. I really don't care, I have been alone all my life and this is no different, but it gives us something to talk about, I guess. Laura wears too much makeup and she uses the wrong color of face powder, which makes her skin very pale. I don't have the courage to tell her she doesn't look real, and I also think that her skin pores can't possibly breathe normally under so much makeup. But I don't have the courage to tell her my worries. She dresses very proper and wears her blonde hair up and twisted into a bun on top of her head in the style of today's fashion. I wear my hair most of the time straight down because curlers give me a headache. When I want the "curly " look I use newspaper strips to curl my hair, it lasts about two hours before it goes straight again. Laura is also very skinny; I don't think that she eats much. She doesn't like school and intends to get married as soon as she is allowed to start dating. Her parents are not making her marry anyone in particular, but they are strict and she is not to date until she is eighteen years old.

A chicken and a turkey disappeared from our backyard. The household is in an uproar, because we don't know who could have stolen them. The police were called, and there were no clues. This means we don't have the main course for New Year's dinner.

Winter of 1959

Papa gave me a book by the American writer, Hemingway. "From now on, you will read only classic books, the kind a young lady should read, quality writing. Your mother told me about the silly girly novels you have been reading. They are no good for you, and put crazy ideas in a young girl's head. When you finish this one you let me know and I'll get you another book."

I was thrilled to have a new book to read. I said thank you and ran into the sunroom to read the first pages.

Mamma mia!!!! I am stunned that Americans are so talented at writing music and yet when it comes to books this is the worst I have ever read. I have been skipping pages as I read this guy's book. Ernest Hemingway has very poor skills at writing, in my personal opinion. He uses little paragraphs, not enough description, and lots of bad words. Talk about trashy stuff! My romantic novel's worst moment is a kiss, which drove Mama nuts. I am not going to say anything; we will see what other books Papa comes up with next. I would rather have books about Egyptian, French, and Portuguese history. I'm going to go bonkers reading this boring *American literature*, as Papa calls it.

Max-Leão was on national television. He was the guest star of the evening talk show, and I was very impressed how he was able to pull through it. Poor thing, he must have been so scared. We never talk about his writing. I feel this is a taboo subject and I don't dare to bring more pressure into his life. He has enough discomfort already inside his ears. Mama keeps saying that Max-Leão is very loving, always on his knees hugging her, but he told me that the reason he is always hugging her that way and putting his head on her lap is because the pressure of her hands over his ears helps to ease the pain. I believe that Mama is aware of that, otherwise why would she press her hands over his ears?

An English woman came to my school; Miss Alexandra something, she was an agent or a scout of some kind trying to find ballerinas for her school in London. She came up to me and as she touched my legs she commented on my strong legs and good posture and she asked me how long I had been dancing and if I wanted to be a professional ballerina. I had to control my emotions when I told her that I would love to be a real ballerina. Either she or the school's principal called Mama that day, because when I got home Mama told me that "No" was the answer; I was not going to England. I am her only daughter and I am too young to be far away from her. I was not surprised; these are not her plans for my life.

This afternoon Max-Leão and I were walking a few blocks from our home on the Avenida Duke de Avila when a group of schoolgirls dressed in their white uniforms saw us. One of them screamed to the others, "It's Max-Leão! It's Max-Leão!" And they came running down the hill towards us.

Max- Leão grabbed my arm and yelled, "Quick, let's run for our lives, they will kill us if they catch us."

We ran like bats out of hell around the street corner and took refuge through an open apartment door facing the street. We locked it from inside and waited a while until the mad group of girls had gone by yelling his name. Finally silence told us it was safe to leave. I wonder what they would have done to him, and to me being his sister, if they had caught him. Being famous can be a curse!

Someone snitched on my brother José. We found out José was the one that kidnapped the chickens and the turkey. He had hidden the birds in his friend's backyard because he didn't want them to be killed. He even paid from his own allowance for their feed and care. Everyone was touched by this act of kindness but that didn't save the chicken and the turkey from their cruel destiny. We ate them, except for José who got away from eating the birds by getting sick with an asthma attack that took him into the hospital. He is now taking experimental drugs to see if they help his asthma.

When I got home today I heard that Max-Leão was doing a science project for school and tried to conduct a science experiment by locking himself in the bathroom and covering all the holes under the door and window so that oxygen couldn't get in. He had made too much smoke by burning some stuff and was discovered just in time. The details are not very clear if he was found unconscious. The whole thing is hush-hush, as with everything that happens in our family. "Max-Leão has no future in Portugal and Israel is not the answer either. He will wind up killed in one of their wars," Mama keeps saying over and over again.

Running Away From the Schoolgirls.

After his second published book, he received a personal letter from the Israel government inviting him to become a citizen and to live there. Mama was horrified with the idea that if he went to Israel he would be nabbed into the military and die with a bullet in his head. Papa is to get in touch with his family in England and to send Max-Leão away as soon as possible.

Papa cracks me up sometimes. When there's no one in the kitchen he sneaks into the refrigerator, takes a raw egg out, puts a pin through it and sucks the egg out, next he carefully puts the empty eggshell back. When Mama or the maid goes to the refrigerator to use the eggs, they can't figure out what happened to them. I am Papa's partner in crime. My job is to stand by the kitchen door and whistle at him if anyone is coming down the hallway. It took months before one evening they caught Papa red-handed, sucking on an egg. He got a real kick out of the whole thing.. I think it's funny too. What's not funny is when he goes into the kitchen to make soup. It doesn't matter if it is instant soup mix, the latest in prepared foods. No "real" man goes into the kitchen to cook. The maid says only queers go in the kitchen, and every time he makes soup the maid giggles and laughs and makes fun of Papa behind his back. Mama finally convinced Papa to make soup only on Sundays, when the maid is off. Most likely the whole neighborhood knows by now that Papa likes to cook.

I know a little now about queer men. Mama explained that they are men that don't like women, only men and boys. They trick young boys into having sex with them by letting them put their penis into their anus, then they wait until the young boys really like having sex that way, then tell them if they want to do it again they have to let them do it to them too. I imagine that it must be very painful, probably as bad as putting the penis into a vagina. She told me also that all queer men have a depraved look about themselves. Many times I have stood on the balcony of my bedroom having fun watching the people in the street go by and I have noticed that the men visiting the queer neighbor next door don't look any different from anybody else. I have a feeling this is another gossip-story that the neighbors and Mama have made up.

Mama asked me to write some poetry, as she wanted to know if I have any talent as a poetess. I got some paper, sat at the desk in my bedroom, and wrote a few scribbles throughout the day.

These few scribbles were given to her at the end of the day: "Do you think that death might be easier than life?" I have wondered about that often enough, and then thinking about love and how lonely I felt I wrote, "I learned to love and then I learned all about suffering." I went on further with my thoughts: "There's only a shadow between the two of us, death, but if you choose to go with me because you love me, then love will conquer death."

After lunch I added, "When we are together, my dream turns to reality, when we are apart, I am left in the abyss of darkness." "How can you curse the stars, that prophesize your own destiny?" "Man is just dust, they say, but I believe they forgot to add that he also has a heart full of dreams and ideals."

For the next one I pulled on all my resources of thought, as I wanted to shock Mama. After all, if Max-Leão's books were all about sex and passion I could do the same: "Give me just one hour in your arms, let me feel the sexual ecstasy of love and then I will leave satisfied because I have learned what is the essence of life itself." I was happy with that one.

Mama took my scribbles with her and came back to my bedroom not long afterwards, saying, "You are definitely not a poetess," and she added, "Don't worry; I'll give them back to you later."

I really tried to write poetry to make her happy, but I couldn't. I'd rather write stories; children's stories and detective stories, the scarier the better.

I don't like poetry because it only expresses what is in the poet's mind, a swirl of thoughts that can be misunderstood or interpreted differently by the reader. I'd rather have straightforward words that say everything in a clear purpose. Poetry is a lot like math; *gumbo, blah, blah*. I hope she throws away what I wrote.

Papa gave me another book for my collection, *The Diary of Anne Frank*. I cried as I read it last night, and before I went to sleep I promised myself to try my best to understand Mama. If either one of us dies or we both die we will never see each other again and I don't want to be like Anne Frank. I don't want to lose Mama. I love her. I just don't understand her. It is so hard for me to connect with her, but I am going to try my very best and be good, the way she wants me to be.

I would love to be an archaeologist, either that or a ballerina, but if I had to choose I would pick archaeologist. Papa gave me a new book, *The Egyptian* by Mika Waltari. This is my very favorite book; once I started reading it I couldn't stop. I have read it twice, and it literally puts me in Egypt.

Papa and Mama have no idea that *The Egyptian* is a real adult book. The main character is a young Egyptian doctor called Sinuhe who falls in love with a beautiful but heartless woman who makes her living by lying down with men. She is only out for one thing, making money. Sinuhe is very angry with her, and in a moment of madness and jealousy he gives her a special concoction that puts her to sleep. He personally takes her to the house of death where they are professionals at taking the guts out and embalming people to be put inside the pyramids, as is the Egyptian custom. But what he didn't foresee is that she woke up before they cut her open, and the men inside the mortuary fell in love with her and wanted her for themselves, so she used the same technique of getting presents from the ones that could afford her. With her charms she not only got away alive, but also very rich because they were all paying for her services. And Sinuhe goes on to describe how he treated the Pharaoh for headaches by drilling a hole into the Pharaoh's skull.

This book is about the strange Egyptian way of life, their old religions and culture. I was reading it last night in the dining room and once again I was so lost into the story that I didn't even notice that it was getting dark in the room or that Papa had walked into the house. He came into the dining room where I was seated with my head basically under the table, as I held the book on my lap and he turned the light on. I didn't expect it and as I lifted my head to look up I hit my nose into the hard wood tabletop. Papa said, "Daughter, you are going to be blind reading in the dark."

He is a good father. The other night I was dozing off to sleep and he walked into my bedroom, and he reached for my blanket and covered my feet, saying in his harsh German accent, "Daughter, you better cover your feet while you sleep, you are going to catch a cold sleeping that way." And he walked away. I don't get hugs or kisses from Mama or Papa but I love and appreciate words that show they care.

What a racket at school today! I sat in the corner of the classroom, looking at the brainless girls in Geometry class. They were crying and crying over some guy in North America who was going to be put to death in the electric chair for killing a couple of girls.

"Imagine," said one of them, hysterically, "the poor man is nothing but a tortured soul, abused as a child by his family, what do you expect?"

I don't care how abused he was as a child. I was happy that he was being executed, but I didn't say anything. They were frantic after reading the story in the Diário de Noticias — most likely it was written by communist writers, who hate Americans and will do anything to make them look like mean selfish capitalists taking over the world, when the truth is that Communists are the ones that want to take over the world. I know that because Mama's brother Uncle Abraham

Reading *The Egyptian*.

is one of them and he doesn't even hide the fact because he never got a proper education and believes anyone with more money than him should share it with him and others less fortunate.

I don't agree with him, because if I had a good job and I worked hard at being successful I'd deserve my paycheck and I should not be forced to share it with someone that is lazy and doesn't want to work or does something else for a living.

Spring of 1959

I got into trouble at school, but I didn't get suspended. That would mean that they would lose my tuition for the month, so I got reprimanded instead. I was never so embarrassed in my life. I got caught during class break playing the paper spin game with a couple of classmates. Every girl my age plays this game. You spin the handmade paper top on a flat surface and if it falls on the number you picked, you open it to unfold the answer to your question, in this case I had written on the inside of the top: *He loves you. He doesn't love you. He wants to kiss you. You want to kiss him. You will be getting married soon.*

I got into trouble for that because I got caught. I never get away with anything, but everybody else does. The principal said she was totally disappointed since she thought that until now I was a very proper and dignified person, but I was nothing more than a silly schoolgirl. Well, I *am* a schoolgirl, darn it. Even my own mother thought it was funny, and when I told her what happened in school she laughed about it.

Big deal indeed; they are lucky that my Cousin Gabriel, doesn't go to their school. He climbed the high school cafeteria wall, nobody knows how he got up there, and broke off the clock's hour arm. Time is standing still in his high school until they repair the old clock on the wall. Cousin Gabriel also likes to inflict pain, and I don't like him. He is a bully. When he comes over our house he likes to pinch me, and then has the nerve to ask, "Does it really hurt? Tell me Verónica, how much does it hurt?" He is fat, has reddish hair, and sweats a lot. King Henry VIII probably looked like him when he was younger. Gabriel is too strong and big for me to fight him off, so when I see him I stay away from him. He wants to be a doctor like his father. The family thinks he is a genius because they found him sewing back a cat's tail that he had previously cut off. "He will probably become a darn good surgeon when he gets older. He has done that several times and is getting good with the stitching," Said Aunt Heydee in admiration of her nephew. Sick little bastard! He is more like a Dr. Frankenstein if anyone asked me.

I heard Mama telling Aunt Heydee during one of her visits to our house how much Mama admires Burt Lancaster's masculinity, and his acting too, of course. She added, "I can't help it if am a romantic, when I met my Joaquim (she doesn't like Papa's German name Hans, so she calls him Joaquim, the Portuguese name for Hans) of course I fell in love with him immediately and I remember fantasizing — you know — he would lure me into his arms and take me somewhere into a little village out in the country, where we could make passionate love."

Up to this point Papa had seemed to be busy reading his newspaper; lifted his head up and said ironically, "Branca, are you telling me that you wanted to have sex with me before marriage?"

Mama didn't expect that question. Papa continued, "If I had known at the time that it was all you wanted, I would have had my way with you and would not have needed to marry you. What a fool I was!" And then he started laughing and so did everybody else.

I wondered if Papa was saying the truth though. Aunt Heydee has told me several times, "Why would the milkman buy a cow, when he can get the milk for free?"

One of the girls in our school who always arrives in her own private chauffeured car has been found to be pregnant and won't be returning to high school. The stories are varied; some think that she was fooling around with her chauffeur because he is the only man that drives her around, and they say the chauffeur is very handsome. Others that knew her personally said it was one of her brother's friends. Either way it doesn't matter; she is going to be a mother, unless she does like Rosa, one of Papa's employers. Rosa is married and has a son but doesn't want anymore children; every time she gets pregnant she goes to a special doctor and aborts the baby. She doesn't even bother to tell her husband.

Mama is looking for a new place for us to spend the summer vacation. This time she wants to try the countryside. It's horrible; I don't like the boring countryside. I prefer the beach. But she says her brother Augusto told her it's good for the nerves and a lot more relaxing. She has taken me along from town to town, checking out houses for rent. There's always something that doesn't meet Mama's requirements; one house is too big, another is too small, another is too expensive, or the owner of another one has sons or a son my age. I always sit quietly on the corner of the room as Mama pleasantly interviews each landlord and their family. This morning she finally found a house that was to her liking, and I sat there listening to her, keeping my fingers crossed that this was the one we would be moving to during the summer.

"So, will you be living close by with your family?" Mama asked her.

"Yes," said the woman with a friendly smile, "Our other house is right around the corner."

Mama was on a mission as she asked with the same caring smile, "How nice. And do you have children?"

"Yes, one very handsome boy, his name is José. As a matter of fact he is your daughter's age. I am sure they are going to get along just great."

As soon as I heard that I knew we were not going to be renting the house from this woman.

When we left I tried to use psychology by asking, "Wasn't the house beautiful and the lady so friendly?"

"Yes, to all that, but I know exactly what you are thinking about," Mama assured me. "You would like to meet her son who is the same age as you, but that is never going to happen."

I hate my mother!

Papa was very surprised with my gift for his birthday, a small diamond pin for his tie. It was a very small diamond, but he acted like it was the biggest diamond in the whole world. He hugged me and his eyes were teary. I could see that he was moved because he said, "Daughter, you are my pride and joy, thank you!"

It was worth saving all my money for a year just to hear him say that.

Today I was taken by surprise when a man in the street corner opened his gabardine and flashed me his private parts while smiling. I stopped and stared at him for a moment because he had no hair down there and I thought that all adults have pubic hair. He stopped smiling and seemed upset that I was more curious than anything else, but my first thought was, *Poor guy, he has a small, defective, pink penis.* He rapidly closed his raincoat, as if suddenly he was ashamed of himself, and walked away from me. I just stood there not knowing if I should yell for the police or ignore the whole thing. I opted for acting like I had not seen anything but when I got home I had to tell someone what had happened and Mama was the first person I saw. She told me that some people are mentally sick and they get a kick out of showing off their sex organs. That is what I call *nuts!*

Tomorrow is my birthday. I am going to be fifteen years old. I have no doubt in my mind that this time there's going to be a surprise birthday party. I wonder what it's going to be like.

It's not everyday that one is fifteen years old; this is a very magical number. Most likely I will get unique presents and a big tall birthday cake and new clothes like the ones Encarnação makes for her daughters, made of taffeta and lace. There will be a lot of colorful balloons decorating the house and I'll get a radio of my own and I will be so happy. My life will be different from now on, because I will be treated like an adult. I am going to sleep now and dream about tomorrow's festivities.

I saw three movies today, the early matinee with Aunt Heydee, midday with Mama, and the evening one with both my parents. Once again nothing different happened. After the usual dinner of codfish boiled with vegetables, the family had the usual rice pudding for dessert and I was given a cupcake with a candle to blow – even though we now can afford a *real* birthday cake – and that was the highlight of the festivities.

There was no dancing or singing, just another uneventful birthday of getting a skirt and blouse that Mama made, that I refuse to wear. The skirt has yellow roses, purple roses, and red roses, all on a vivid green background. Anyone can see me from miles away. And then to add insult to injury she also made, from the same ugly material, an ornamental pin that is supposed to look like a rose to be attached to my new orange and purple shirt. I'd rather die than be seen in an outfit like that. I know that I hurt her feelings, but the gaudy rose pin she made with tiny balls hanging out of it, is beyond anything I can possibly endure.

Max-Leão heard me crying in my bedroom and sat next to me on my bed saying he didn't know why I was crying when I had gotten such an original and beautiful outfit. He likes it so much that he wants me to wear it when we go out together so that everybody thinks that I am his girlfriend. He was trying to make me feel better, but it didn't help. Mama probably told him what to say.

I am going to sleep tonight and freeze myself in a cocoon covered with bricks, completely sealed from the outside world, and I will stay this way as a fifteen year old until the day that I am an adult and happy; only then will I come out and start living again.

I will never again try to cheat in school. It was a waste of time, not to mention my nerves were shot worrying that I would get caught. For the geography test I wrote some of the main rivers of Portugal on the left palm of my hand and for the algebra class I wrote some of the basic ideas on the palm of my right hand. I have trouble memorizing. I have the brain of a bird, a small bird most likely. But I was so scared that I would be caught that I didn't even have the courage to open my hands while taking the tests. Afterwards I ran to the bathroom to wash the ink off the palms of my hands and realized that nothing I had written, not even one of them was the answer to any of the questions. If I had been caught I would have been harshly punished for nothing.

I love dreaming about love. I do that whenever I feel lonely; like before falling asleep, when I am sitting at a coffee shop, and even in school. I look straight at the teacher and don't even see her. I look straight past her and into my own world. It's amazing how much I can hide by looking like I am paying attention and yet — I am not even there.

In my big mansion there are guests staying overnight. I can't sleep; it's a very hot and humid summer night. Dressed in my long, silk, yellow gown I walk downstairs and open the French doors to the garden. A light breeze caresses my body as I breathe deep into my lungs the pure oxygen of the mountains around me, when suddenly I feel that he is there: the man I love. I don't know if he really loves me, and we have hardly had a chance to talk since the party last night. My parents kept me busy in the kitchen helping prepare dinner. I know he is there because he can't sleep either, because he was thinking about me, and he would like to kiss me. The flicker of his cigarette lighter is on as he approaches me.

"Cigarette?"

"You are so beautiful," he says as he comes closer to me.

I am in a trance; I can smell his aftershave cologne. The soft breeze gives me a chill.

"You are cold," he says as he puts his cigarette out. "Let me put my arms around you."

He holds me by the waist and then, very softly, his hand moves away the small hair-curl that has fallen over my face. His hand caresses me ever so softly. His face is very close to mine and our lips meet for the first time. It is a passionate kiss, just like in the novels I have read.

Sometimes my lover and I meet at a dance, at someone's house, or even in the street, but the happy ending is always the same, with a kiss of love. My lover has no real face. He is a love spirit created out of my loneliness. Nobody knows about my made-up lover.

My favorite subject in school is English. I love History and Ballet, but English is like sunshine, happiness, ice cream, and strawberries! I melt in the English language! *Love*, what a word! *Kiss*, another word for lips and touching. *Moon*, the dark nights are lit by the *moonlight* while two lovers *kiss* in *love*. *Chewing gum*, *America*, *cigarettes*, *Oklahoma* where the cowboys meet the girls and everyone is happy singing and dancing until they fall in love and get married and live happily ever after.

Summer of 1959

Horror of horrors! I made the mistake of not wearing underwear when I went out today. It's Aunt Heydee's fault. She is always bragging that during the hot summer months she doesn't wear underwear, that way she keeps cool when she walks outside. So I tried it too. My luck; as I was almost home, right in front of our front door, while I was waiting for the downstairs door to open after I pressed the buzzer, a strong gust of wind came towards me and swirled my wide skirt up. I was naked to the world as all the men and women, passing by stared at me smirking. Now they know where I live. I hope nobody saw my face. I am not going out for a few days.

Aunt Heydee is a very petite woman who has been shrinking as she gets older. She is old but still very beautiful. She has big green eyes and her smooth light skin compliments her blonde hair, which looks very natural. Her beauty secret is the daily use of almond oil on her skin, washing her breasts with cold water every morning to keep them from sagging, and using lemons for helping maintain the blonde hair color. She puts fresh lemon juice on her hair and once in a while she uses peroxide to lighten it even more; the sun always helps to speed up the process. Her special title of "Napoleão #1" is very befitting; everybody agrees that if she had been born a man she would have conquered the world. I admire her tenacity more than anything else. Anything she puts her mind to, she does it, and nothing is impossible for her. Her age is not important since there's no way she is going to tell us, and if she were to tell us, we would learn only that she is older than what she was thirty years ago. Therefore it is simpler to say that this story happened a few years back in the past, somewhere in time:

One day, Aunt Heydee was looking through the newspaper and read an announcement that President Salazar would be a guest during a big political function. It was going to be the event of the year, the ball of your dreams, dancing most likely to waltz-type of music, chatting and flirting with some of the top-notch men in government, mixing in with royalty, eating caviar, and drinking bubbling champagne from crystal glasses. Aunt Heydee decided that she was going to attend the event. It didn't matter that she had not been invited. The only apparent difficulty was to find something to wear that would fit the royal occasion. She only had plain clothes; basically clothes that were more like Cinderella's wardrobe before she married the prince.

So, Aunt Heydee was seated in her dining room feeling sad when suddenly, upon looking up, she noticed how splendid the old golden brocade curtains hanging in the window looked. Yes, they were old and dusty but their possibilities were left to the imagination, and *that* she had a lot of.

She asked Grandma Rica, her mother, if she could borrow the curtains for the evening, and went right into the old Singer sewing machine where, in a jiffy, a masterpiece was created. A few golden ropes here and there, no one was even going to dream she was wearing her curtains.

She took the trolley car as far as she could and then, around the corner from the Palácio de Queluz, she picked up a taxi for her grand entrance. A doorman awaited the arrival of the evening guests, and when she entered the man at the door dressed in red and gold uniform simply asked, "Madam, gold or silver invitation?"

"Gold, of course," she said without blinking an eye, and wearing a glorious smile. No one dared to question her as to whether she actually had an invitation with her. She looked like royalty. The handsome man at the door was more than happy to offer her his arm and took her personally to the "gold room" where she spent the evening dancing and talking to everyone she met. And yes, she danced with the vice-president of Portugal, only because the president was not able to attend the soiree.

We are spending the summer in a little town called Malveira. I don't know why we are staying here when Mama said a few times already that the name of the town is like a curse name of bad things to come because it reminds her of "maldição," the Portuguese word for curse. Malveira is very isolated, and the only fun thing to do is to walk to the so-called town — which is a street with a grocery store and a coffee shop, that's it.

At night, Max-Leão, José and I stand at the window in the hallway upstairs and we look outside trying to spot a werewolf, a witch, or even a ghost. Anything scary would bring some excitement into our lives. After we get tired and sleepy from looking into the dark woods that surround us we

Aunt Heydee.

each go to our bedrooms. Most of the time, I'll sit on my bed and read Portuguese history books. I love reading Portuguese history in this old house; it fits the house we live in; old and dark and in the middle of nowhere.

In this forsaken place I only have two choices to keep me from going insane: reading or writing, there's nothing else to do here. In Costa da Caparica or Eiriceira I could walk along the shore or take a walk through their villages and hang out by one of their coffee shops at the center of town where the residents sit and watch the tourists go by. There are no tourists around here; we are the only city people. I am not allowed to walk alone into the woods around Malveira, or go up one of the hills in the distance, and much less into the quarry where I went a few times to play with stones. Mama told me that last week a girl was raped in the woods and then dragged to the quarry where no one could hear her scream for help. She had been found dead. The police are still looking for the criminal. I don't know what to do except read and write. But I get tired of sitting because my tailbone hurts from all these hard wooden chairs.

So, this week I dared Max-Leão to take a walk with me on the highway. I dared him to see how far we could walk from where we live. We walked all morning, and when the sun came up on us like a burning oven we didn't stop, we were going to walk as far as the other side of the world. By the end of the day our feet were killing us and we knew we couldn't make it back home. We were exhausted when we stopped at the next town's tavern. They let us use their telephone to call home to see if someone could pick us up. Nope, no one was going to come and get us, and we were told to walk back home. The bartender felt sorry for us and drove us back in his car. It was a miracle that he felt sorry for us.

After this experience, the idea of running away for me is gone, at least not by trying to walk as far as I can. You can only go a couple of miles and your feet start to kill you, not to say anything about nighttime, when it's cold and the wolves are roaming the fields. I should have learned from Mama a few years back when she used to hit me a lot, and one day she was really angry and grabbed me by the hair and pulled me down the hallway to the front door. She opened the door and said, "Get out of this house now. I don't want you here anymore!" I cried and cried, mostly because while I was crying I was thinking, *I can never leave because I have no place to go, and she knows that.*

Aunt Heydee was visiting us for the weekend, so I decided to unveil the beginnings of my first detective story to her and Mama. I invited them both to the only coffee shop down the road from us, where my inspiration had grown out of complete solitude and boredom.

I took a good look at them and prepared them by saying, "Be ready to get startled by detailed descriptions of crime scenes."

I immediately started to read the first page.

"It was a dark night, as dark as the deepest well made by the devil himself. Detective Peter Smith tried holding his breath as the sewage stink crept up his nostrils and filled his lungs. His tall skinny body was literally covered by the oversized gray gabardine which made him almost invisible as he walked firmly through the thick fog, which seemed to be there just to blind him without mercy. Slapping his wet muddy shoes through this narrow slum street of London, a rat ran between his feet...

"Stop!" Mama cried out, "What a heavy, depressing ghastly story for a young girl to write. I can't stand it; your writing is going to give me nightmares. You should be writing about love, not about dreadful things like crime, and who knows what you wrote on the next pages."

"You don't want to hear the rest of my detective story?" I asked, knowing well in advance that I had hit a nerve.

"No," said Mama getting up from her chair, "I've heard enough."

Aunt Heydee didn't say much, only winked an eye at me but before we all left the coffee house she whispered in my ear, "Don't stop writing even if people think it's too morbid. You are the writer and you are Napoleão #2, don't forget that."

I had cut deep into their minds, and the person I mostly wanted to stir was Mama. So what, she didn't like my writing. I was not surprised by her reaction. Impressing her with a story, even if it was a sinister one, was for me a great accomplishment.

As always after lunch, everybody goes into their bedroom to take a nap. I don't like napping so I have kept busy, taking a fast twenty-minute walk as I breathe in slowly and deep the awesome smell of the eucalyptus field I cross in order to reach the coffee shop in town. I don't even know why it is called a town; maybe because the houses are closer to each other along the highway. It's a real small, dinky coffee shop that doubles as a tavern. The place is big enough for four very small, round, wood tables with two hard wooden chairs each. There are no windows; the light that comes in is filtered through the beads hanging from the top of the two entrances. There are no signs like "in" or "out," but you know that one doorway is to come in and the other is to go out. I learn things like these from watching the customers. I am there every day, sitting at my usual small, round, wood table by the entrance, acting all grown up with a cup of coffee next to me, writing my detective story and sipping the coffee ever so slowly so that it will last for hours.

Three boys about my age walked into the coffee shop. One of them turned out to be a real jerk. He seemed normal until his eyes met mine.

"What do we have here?" he said, putting his hand to his chest. "A flower in the middle of an oasis?" And he pointed at me, as if he had found a treasure that I was not aware of. The other two boys were laughing at him, as the young fool acted as if he had just seen the love of his life. He threw himself on the floor and then dramatically got up and banged his body into the front of the wood counter where the owner stood while staring at the theatrical madness not quite understanding what it was all about. "I want her to be my wife," said the kid, once again putting his hand over his chest as if he was having a heart attack. "I am in love! I am in love! I am in love!" he kept screaming as if he was out of his mind. His friends were laughing while they were trying to restrain him.

I felt embarrassed and also scared, picked up my papers, and was ready to leave when the owner put his hand firmly on my shoulder. "No, you stay. They are the ones leaving now, or I'll break all three necks with my bare hands."

They left, dragging the crazy boy with them. I waited a while for the coast to be clear, and then I went home. I was never so humiliated in my life. I know that I am just an average girl, and for this boy to put on such a stupid act was an insult. He was definitely making fun of me. Now I feel ugly and very sad.

A letter arrived today. It's from the boy I met at the coffee shop. He asks Mama to allow him to visit me and that he would like to apologize for his behavior towards me and would like to be my boyfriend. As if that wasn't enough, he went on saying that he couldn't forget me since he saw me. I can't forget him either, how can one forget somebody that embarrassing.

Mama asked Max-Leão if he knew the boy, he did and had been meaning to tell us today that Artur, who lives up on the hill, is very rich — well, at least his parents are very rich and they have a huge swimming pool on their property. Max-Leão knows Artur, they are acquaintances, and yesterday when they were talking, Artur found out that Max-Leão is my brother and he invited Max-Leão to come for a swim in his pool.

Mama told me not to worry about the crazy kid on the hill. She would answer his letter not only to him but also to his family in a way that would stop him from ever bothering me again.

Max-Leão wouldn't stop teasing me, making me feel guilty. I am depriving him of swimming in Artur's swimming pool in the hot summer days ahead. I don't care if he is rich and has a pool, I am not going to sacrifice myself like a virgin on a mountain of fire so that Max-Leão can keep cool this summer. Besides, Mama is on my side this time. When she finishes writing a letter to him and his family I am sure that he will feel like I do, miserable.

I don't know what to think. I am very scared. Aunt Heydee called us this morning to tell us that our parents are both in the hospital. They were on their way here from Lisbon when a car hit Papa's motorcycle from behind. They were both thrown off the motorcycle. Mama is in a coma and might die. I have been praying for them. *Please dear God don't let my parents die.* I can't stand this thought.

Papa came home; he has lots of bruises all over his face. He called me to his side and said in a very weary voice, "My daughter, from now on you are in charge of the household. This is the amount of money I gave your mother every month. You are to pay the bills and oversee the maid and handle what meals are to be served daily,"
"I want to see Mama," I said assertively.
"She can't have visitors, but you being the eldest I guess you have that right. Your brothers will have to stay here. I will take you with me tomorrow morning to the hospital, but you will have to come back alone, by bus. I have to stay in Lisbon because of work at the office and I don't want to leave Mama alone at night."
I could see that he was tired and thinking out loud as he said once again, "As the eldest, I guess you have the right to see your mother." And he cried. I cried too with Max-Leão and José. We don't want to be orphans.

It was weird to see Mama lying in a hospital bed, unconscious. She was bruised all over and her head was covered with bandages and she had a cast on her broken leg and another on her broken arm. Aunt Heydee explained that Mama had been thrown from the motorcycle and rolled about 20 meters before going into a ditch. She had hit her head several times along the way. She was bleeding inside from concussions to the brain. Nothing could be done for her. Papa encouraged me to go back to Malveira that day, but I insisted on staying the night with Mama, which allowed Papa to go home and get some sleep. He thanked me for it and showed me the straight armchair where he had been spending the nights. If by any chance Mama was to wake up from her coma I was to run immediately to the front desk and get a nurse. Mama is in a private room and that's why they allow a family member to stay the night.

I found out that I couldn't sleep seated. It felt like the longest night of my life. Every time I dozed off my neck would be hurting as well as my stiff back. Daylight finally came through the window shades and I got up from my chair of torture. Mama didn't wake up; she was still in a coma, but she was breathing so I decided to take a quick look around the hospital. I left her room and went down the hallway and up and down some stairs looking for a door that would open to somewhere, not really knowing what I was looking for. I saw a door; I opened it and walked in carefully. A man was lying down in a white metal bed, just like Mama. He saw me and said, "Hello, come on in."

I got scared and ran out; as I heard him pleading, "Please don't go. I won't bite; come back!" I went back to Mama's room feeling guilty for being so nosey. He could have been the criminal from Malveira that everybody was looking for, or even worse, a dead man lying on the hospital bed, waiting to be buried. I get goose bumps just thinking about it.

I took the bus back from Lisbon to Malveira. A boy sat next to me. I was nervous, since I rarely have someone of the opposite sex and about my age sitting next to me. I could tell my face was going red and I didn't have anything with me like a book that I could stare at, so I stared out of the window the whole time. But it was a long trip, so I got my potato chips bag and, before I took a chip out, I nervously offered him some. He said politely, "No thank you." He wouldn't look at me either. I could tell that he was as uncomfortable as I was. One stop before Malveira he got up, took a look straight at me, smiled, and left the bus. I took a deep breath of relief, but before the bus took off he rushed back into the bus and very shyly handed me a piece of paper. I wasn't going to read it, that's for sure. I was worried that it might be his name, telephone number, or say something silly like he liked me, or that I was ugly and he hated potato chips. I was afraid to find out. Whatever he had written I was afraid to find out. I opened the window and as the bus took off I threw the still-folded little note out of the window.

Now I feel retarded for having done that, but I would have died of embarrassment if he had asked me to be his girlfriend.

Something weird happened in Malveira while I was visiting Mama in the hospital. The night that I was away, our house got broken into. In the morning the maid found Max-Leão in bed with his legs tied and his hands also tied behind his back, his mouth was taped and bound. It was too dark for him to see the assaulters, and they had blindfolded him before he had a chance to recognize anyone. The dresser drawer in his bedroom had been pulled apart as well as the ones in my bedroom. Someone had been looking for something last night. José and the maid slept through the whole thing. I think they were robbers, but Max-Leão, José and the maid think it was probably the crazy kid from the hill looking for the love letter he sent me. Nothing was missing. I am so lucky that I wasn't home last night.

Until we get back to Lisbon at the end of the month, I am going to lock my bedroom door from the inside, and every night I will push my dresser against the door with all my books on top of it. A robber will not be able to come in without making lots of noise which would wake me up in time to scream loud enough to wake up everybody at home.

We have been eating like kings every day. I told Isabel, our maid, that while Mama is in the hospital, we want fried potatoes for lunch and dinner. The little birds Max-Leão and José catch outside with their slings are to be fried and served that day, if we don't have enough birds we will have steaks instead. We don't want vegetables, but freshly made tomato sauce with sliced onions is a must at every meal, and green soup is welcome everyday for dinner. For breakfast I asked Isabel to make coffee with lots of milk, a soft-boiled egg, and rustic bread with butter and cheese. Midday between lunch and dinner we have a tall glass of milk with coffee and we put bread into it, mash it with a spoon, and add lots of sugar until it turns into a tasty, soggy sweet coffee cake.

Mama is no longer in a coma and she should be here with us in a month, about the time we are going back to Lisbon. I can't wait for Mama to come home. She is going to be so proud of me when I give her the money I have saved while she was in the hospital. Papa gave me too much money to run the household.

Mama came home but she is still very sick. She lost a lot of weight and she faints all the time. She needs a lot of silence around her, otherwise the headaches get worse.

Mama thanked me for giving her the money I saved while she was in the hospital and asked me not to tell Papa about it, otherwise he will give her less money each month and this is the money she uses for buying us special goodies or anything she needs without having to beg for extra cash. She added, "I am going to teach you how to budget a household and save money from what your husband gives you every month. It's always a good idea to have a little extra for a rainy day. All smart women prepare for the future by having a little nest-egg saved."

Autumn of 1959

When girls become women they bleed, and when boys become men they have to get initiated into manhood by going to the house of prostitution to learn about having sex with women that do that for a living. I don't know which is worse; probably bleeding because you also get belly cramps with it. Max-Leão was given some money and sent to the house of prostitution as a fourteenth birthday present from our parents.

Aunt Heydee, Mama and I waited for him to come home and tell us all about it, we were all curious. I don't know if Papa is really aware of all this since he was not with us waiting for my brother to come home.

Max-Leão came home about four in the afternoon; he had been gone for over three hours. "Tell us all about it," was the instruction. He mumbled something about a naked woman lying in bed asking him to take his clothes off and to join her. At that point I was asked to leave the room and no matter how much I begged to stay Mama sent me out of the room.

Mama has pain all over her body and her bruises have not healed yet. She is most happy when my brothers and I take turns pushing a wire in and out of her leg cast; that's the only way she can stand the itching.

Mama told me a secret that I am not supposed to tell anyone, or people might think she has gone crazy. She saw Jesus when she was in the hospital. He sat on her bed and talked to her. He was very nice and soothing and held her hand. He sat on her bed, kept her company, and gave her hope for the future.

I think Mama is having stronger hallucinations after getting hit in the head.

Lucia, a Brazilian girl joined our class last month. There were bets that she would never be able to catch up with us because Brazilians are not as smart as Portuguese, and their education is not up to our high standards. But she has not only caught up to us, she passes all tests with high honors. She is very quiet and hardly speaks to anyone. I admire Lucia mostly for being able to live with her cracked lips. They are chapped badly from the cold but she won't bite the skin off. It's amazing to me that she has such self-control where a skin is hanging out her bottom lip and she won't pull it off with her teeth.

One of the girls in class must have felt the same because I heard her going up to Lucia and saying, "Lucia, how can you stand your lips that way, why don't you peel them?"

"It doesn't bother me." And Lucia went back to reading the book on her desk. What a geek!

Mama has to live in complete silence. She can't even listen to music anymore because of horrible headaches. They are so strong that she faints from the pain. This happens three and four times a day since the accident this summer. Even though she got a head concussion and they were afraid that she wasn't going to live because she was in a coma for three weeks, the doctors are now saying, "It's all nerves and in her head and she has a hysterical personality."

Of course it is in her head, theirs would hurt too if they had hit their head on several rocks after rolling on the hard ground about 20 meters from the motorcycle. Anybody would be in pain for a long time if it had happened to him or her.

So they give her "medicine" to calm her down and to sleep. These drugs are a lot more potent than what she used to take before the accident. Mama keeps them in a large shoebox that she carries under her arm from room to room so she doesn't have to walk far to get to them. Her brother, cousins, and personal doctor give all these medicines to help her stay without pain. Mama's leg has not healed properly and it's weak; she must have broken her foot also, because it doesn't work right; she trips a lot over her own feet. She also has gained a lot more weight since she came home. She hurts all over. She has told me that since the accident she has developed sensitive spots all over her body.

Mama was very touched by my birthday present, she even cried from joy. She was born on December 15, but she celebrates her birthday December 5, because she is used to it. December 5 was the date of my grandmother's firstborn. As a memory and respect for the dead baby, her parents changed Mama's birthday to the 5th. I think that was a horrible thing to do, and I don't understand the reasoning, but I have never said anything about it. Mama seems to be perfectly happy with December 5 being her birth date. I gave Mama a beautiful gold pin designed to look like a basket filled with little flowers made of small colorful precious stones. She was very impressed that I had been able to save all my money to buy her the pin. I feel so good about myself. I feel like I can do anything and nothing is impossible as long as I put my mind to it. I like making my parents happy.

Max-Leão and José are jealous of me because Mama gave me her radio for Chanukah. It pays to be the eldest. I get priority on inheritance gifts. My brothers like music, but Mama knows that I *love* music. José is into Geometry and Math, Max-Leão is into cars, and I am the music lover. The radio is to be used only in my bedroom, which is now up front facing the street. If Mama is home, I have to listen to music very low, but that's okay. At least I have music, rock and roll music. American music is the best music in the world.

I am so lucky that I was not riding with Papa on his motorcycle the day they got hit. I would have died, of that I am sure. Like Aunt Heydee said, Mama was lucky to be heavy, because it kept her from rolling even further into the distance. If it had been me, being that I am lighter, I would have rolled into the next town like a cannonball at one hundred kilometers an hour. At one hundred kilometers an hour is how fast they got hit. It's a miracle that both my parents survived.

Winter of 1960

Mama sleeps in the furthest room of the house, away from noise and light, next to the bathroom and the kitchen. The city noises at night keep her awake. I love the sounds of the city; cars honking, brakes trying to stop in time before the cars plow into each other, and if no one really gets hurt you can hear the drivers cursing at each other, blaming one another. A lot of times the police have to intervene or the two motorists will kill each other in hand-to-hand combat. This happens about three to four times a year right around the street corner from where we live. It's a tricky corner and the hill is steep and when you get to the top of the street it's hard to see the coming traffic in either direction. Many pedestrians have been injured or killed while crossing it, since cars have the right of way. I usually walk to the next corner and then cross to the other side. I never play with fate by crossing straight across. When Max-Leão and I were kids we tried a few times sitting on this street corner to see at first hand two cars crashing into each other, but it never happened while we waited, it was always after we had left the site.

Besides hearing the sounds of the traffic outside, I also hear when the garbage men come by our street. They like to throw the empty metal cans back onto the cobblestones. They make enough noise to wake up the dead, but it lets me know I still have two more hours of sleep before I have to get up to go to school. I can also hear the neighbors screaming, so I know who is fighting with whom, and it's usually the couple straight across from my bedroom window. Most of their fights are due to the wife's jealousy. She is constantly accusing her husband of cheating on her as he walks in late at night drunk. He punches her around, but she doesn't leave him. I don't understand her.

The lights from the cars going by hit my bedroom window like flashlights on a dark road; they make all kinds of light designs on the bedroom walls and ceiling. I love my bedroom, and I love my radio and listening to American rock and roll, the new music that has developed in the last few years, but I also have a weakness for Bach.

Aunt Heydee says that Bach is one of the most difficult classical composers to understand and appreciate and she can't believe that I like him. But I do, it sounds like rock and roll music to me, in a classical way. I tried to explain that to her but she didn't believe me. Nobody really understands me. I don't like Portuguese music, the *fado* has no beat and it is depressing. Bach and American music make me happy.

I have to be very careful when holding on to Mama's arm. When we go out to the movies, I am very careful so she doesn't get sore from the pressure. Since the motorcycle accident she seems different, she goes deep into thought, as if she is meditating, on the other hand she takes me with her when she goes out, and she is a lot nicer to me now. I love going out with her, slipping my arm around hers, it feels so warm on a cold winter day. I feel close to her that way. She can't walk too far, one block and she starts to hurt all over. It's also hard on her legs, she walks slowly now, not like she used to. We take taxis every time we go out. The insurance will pay for it when they give her the financial settlement for the pain and suffering she is going through. That's what the lawyer my parents hired to represent Mama, has told them.

What a day! Mama took me to a French beauty shop in downtown Lisbon. It is the most chic beauty shop in all of Lisbon, probably in all of Portugal. Only rich people; foreigners, and probably movie stars go there, it is *that* expensive. She asked for their best stylist, she wanted to see what could be done to make me look better.

A very tall skinny young man with oily hair and the body movements of a ballerina looked at me as if I was some jungle animal that had been forgotten by time. He grabbed my face and pulled at my hair in different directions. His little brown eyes were shining with glee when he asked Mama, "Can I do anything I want with her?"

"Yes, by all means."

He took me into a private room and told two girls as he tossed them some nail coloring, "You already know what I want her nails to look like."

They must have read his mind. One got on her knees, grabbed my feet, took my shoes off, and put my feet into a container with hot sudsy water while the other pulled a chair next to me and started working on my hands.

He returned later, looked over my nails approvingly, and clicked his fingers at me — as if I was a dog — to follow him. He pointed to a chair in front of a mirror. He then turned my chair around with my back to the mirror. He cut and cut and brushed and then he clicked his fingers again, speaking like a broken record, "Makeup! Makeup!"

The same two girls brought him a box of colors. He painted my face. I still had no idea what he was doing to me, and then he called Mama into the room.

"Oh, my God," Mama said as she entered the room, "Verónica, you look like Cleopatra!"

He turned me to the mirror. *Mamma mia*, was that me? With green eye shadow and red lipstick and hair like — I just didn't know what to think. I didn't know that I could look this different. I don't know how much Mama paid for all that work, but it must have been a small fortune.

We left the beauty salon, and as we walked the street people were turning to look at me. I felt funny, not comfortable. We took the trolley and a man looked up and said, "Cleopatra for sure."

Mama was not happy about that remark, "This is going too far, it's going to go to your head. I don't want you to think that you are going to look like this tomorrow, enjoy it for today."

Then another man came into the trolley and, looking straight at me, said in the very typical honest Portuguese

The Beauty Salon.

way, "Very beautiful, but what's a young girl like you wearing all that makeup for? You don't need all that garbage!"

That did it to me. I was out of place. I knew it! I knew it; that's why everybody was looking at me. I don't want to look like someone else, not even Cleopatra.

When we got home, Mama was very straightforward as she told me, "Go into the bathroom and wash your face with soap, then get your hair wet and parted to the side, the normal way, before Papa gets home."

I was glad to do that. I don't ever want to be someone else. Thank God, I am myself again.

Max-Leão and I have reached some maturity, because Mama now allows us both to go dancing on weekends at the Jewish Center. She had two dresses made for me from the fashion magazine the seamstress brought with her. I picked a light blue material and picked the model that looked closest to Audrey Hepburn. She was wearing a simple dress with a round white collar and long sleeves with white cuffs to match.

Mama said she was disappointed in my choice. In her opinion it was a boring dress that didn't do anything for me. But I'd felt it did a lot for me, and it was the look I wanted. The other dress was her choice, purples and blues and fringes and ruffles. When I wore it people commented that I looked like Sophia Loren, but I would rather look like Audrey Hepburn. Now I have three outfits in my wardrobe; the loud outfit with roses that Mama made for me, the sexy Sophia with the low-cut ruffled top, and my favorite — the Audrey look — which is the only one I will always wear to go dancing with Max- Leão.

When I walk in the streets I get a line of cars following me. It's like a curse. I feel like Cousin Esther. I admit that I like it because it means that these men must think that I am pretty enough to follow me, but I don't like it because I know that what they want is sex. They don't know me and they don't love me, so I get mixed feelings about it; I feel like a real woman, but abused to a certain extent. They each slow down, put their head out of the window, and invite me for a ride. Big deal, they have a car. Do they really believe that I am going to go with strangers so that I can be squeezed like a lemon? They cause traffic jams by slowing down the traffic, and when one gives up following me, another one takes over.

I told Aunt Heydee that when I go out I get pinched in crowded areas, and on the trolley or bus they press themselves onto me and I can feel their hard private parts. The other day, a young priest put his hand on top of my hand when I was holding onto the bus railing, so I would not fall when they go for the breaks abruptly or around the street corners at full speed. I thought it might've been my imagination, so I moved my hand but his hand followed right after mine. I left the bus at the next stop and walked home. Aunt Heydee was not sympathetic with my misfortune and she said, "Priests are human beings like you and me and most of all they are men. Imagine a man without a woman to love, that's loneliness!"

Aunt Heydee has an incredible amount of unlimited compassion for everybody. I will never forget the day she took me to a movie matinee and the man seated behind us slipped his hand through the seats and put his hand softly on one of her breasts. She whispered to me, "There's a guy behind my seat and he got his hand over my breast; the poor thing whoever he is, I hope that touching my breast brings him comfort."

I was appalled by her way of thinking, "My goodness, Aunt Heydee, pull his hand off!"

"I can't do that. He probably doesn't have anyone special in his life; besides, he is barely touching me. If this brings him happiness let him enjoy it."

I don't understand Aunt Heydee in these matters. She is too nice; I would have picked up the man's hand and bitten hard.

I tried using the pity act the other day and that worked, but it took a lot out of me to do it. I was riding the trolley during the rush hour, it was jam-packed with passengers, and some guy kept rubbing himself on me. I could feel his private part against my back, so I took a deep breath of courage and yelled out, pointing at him, "This man is squeezing himself against me and touching me in an indecent manner. Can someone help me?"

Two good Samaritans grabbed the molester by his coat and threw him out of the moving trolley before he could even utter a word.

It's been okay to go dancing on Friday nights at the Jewish Center with Max-Leão. But there aren't that many boys attending, and the ones that show up are boring squares. I dance with whoever is available and dream about my future boyfriend, the one that will come my way some day. The best part of our night out is on the way home when Max-Leão and I take our sweet time walking. As long as we are back home by eleven o'clock, our parents don't really care what we do. So on the way home, we stop by the main road being worked on during the day, climb the mounds of sand to the very top, and then slide down trying to stand up while doing that as if we are skiing. Sometimes we throw a couple of *centavos* on the railway to see how flat they get after the trolley drives over them.

About a month ago, a new boy came to the dance. He was tall, slim, and knew how to dance, a rarity in itself. While dancing, I tried not to look at him because his face was ugly with pockmarks, but still he was the best looking of them all. He always asked me to dance with him, but we never talked. I didn't know what to say and he didn't have anything to say either, I guess. I have not seen him for the last two weekends; probably his family moved out of Portugal. I don't know his name. We didn't have anything in common that I was aware of except that we danced really well together.

243

~ *Chapter Six* ~

The Spanish Letters

1960

Spring of 1960

Mama gave me a large safety pin. A girl's best friend is a safety pin, she told me, and it works great in crowds of any type. No one comes near me anymore; well, they do, but they immediately move away when I stab their legs with it.

Aunt Heydee is my best friend, my only friend. I still visit Encarnação as often as I can, but she never goes out, she is home all the time. Aunt Heydee is "hip." She is young at heart. She laughs and says silly things, and she always says something that makes me think, and has meaning about life. She takes me to the coffee shops downtown and we get to sit at the most sophisticated for hours watching the people go by. It's a lot of fun. She always makes friends with whoever is sitting close to us, most of the time people from other countries, tourists. She speaks so many languages that she can talk to any tourist.

Yesterday she made me laugh because of the way she went up to the trolley car driver and asked him to go faster or we would be late for an important appointment. She didn't dare to tell him we were only trying to get downtown faster. When he said he could only drive the speed limit, she slipped 25 *centavos* into his hand as if she was giving him a million *centavos,* and smiled at him with all her charm. He speeded

245

down the hill and down the avenue, ringing the bell all the way to our destination: the movie theatre.

Mama has been writing a lot of poetry since her accident. She writes every day. She carries paper with her and a pen, and she is constantly busy writing. Papa says that the bump on Mama's head has awakened her artistic vein. She writes a lot and everybody loves her poetry. Aunt Heydee believes that Mama should publish her works. I have tried to understand what she writes, but to me it's just something else about her that I don't understand. Her poetry is all about sexual innuendos and doesn't rhyme. I have come to the conclusion that I simply don't like poetry.

This morning we all went to the airport to wait for Aunt Nelly. She is Mama's sister from North America. It was nice to see the whole family together and in an excited uproar when Nelly came down the steps from the plane. We were cheering and yelling her name, all excited to see her. She looked like she did in her pictures except that she was bigger, I mean stocky, but not fat. I hugged her and she kissed me and I liked her immediately because she smiled a lot and kept kissing me and hugging me as if I was special in her life. She smelled like Wrigley's Juicy Fruit chewing gum. I heard Mama whispering to Aunt Heydee, "What do you think happened to her arms? They are so wide!"

Aunt Nelly was very tired and barely touched the special dinner we made for her, boiled chicken covered with homemade mayonnaise and a side vegetable salad with mayonnaise dressing. Only the soup was normal, collard green soup, my favorite. The use of mayonnaise and chicken is only for special occasions like holidays or when we are trying to impress someone. This dinner was very expensive, something we really can't afford daily, but it was a special occasion and we were obviously trying our best to impress her with the French cuisine. Nelly hardly ate anything. She said she was getting nauseous and got excused from the table and retired early to bed. It was very disappointing.

We were all up early today to hear more from Aunt Nelly. She told us she didn't like mayonnaise, it made her nauseous. Poor thing, no wonder she was feeling sick last night with dinner. She had a box of chocolate mints and shared it with all of us. She let me choose a pair of earrings from her personal jewelry box. I chose the silver earrings with the light blue stones. They are small and delicate, that would be something Audrey Hepburn would have used in one of her movies. I can't believe that Aunt Nelly is so kind and so very giving. Everything about her is North American. Even when she speaks Portuguese, she has an American accent. We are all so lucky to have someone like her visiting us, all the way from North America, a country full of millionaires, cowboys and Indians, New York City and Hollywood, and she is my aunt, and she treats me like an adult. It's incredible!

Aunt Nelly is interested in talking to me and whenever she goes anywhere, she wants me to go with her. She hugs me and kisses me as if we have always known each other. I love listening to her talk about life in North America.

This afternoon we all sat on Nelly's bed as she told us about her hard times. In the wintertime, she had to shovel coal under her house in order to heat it up, if we could even imagine so much snow outside.

I have only seen snow once. I remember because I was at Grandma's house, and when I looked outside the window I saw snow for the first time in my life, white chunky fluffy ice falling out of the sky. I remember my hands freezing until they were numb as I kept them outside the window.

Snow tastes like sorbet without fruit flavor. I had to walk home that afternoon and I kept making little balls of snow and eating them, then my hands and tongue got so cold that I had to stop until they got warm again. It wasn't a lot of snow falling, but it was enough for the motorists to get out of their cars and scrape enough snowflakes to make silly fun things on top of their cars' roof and then drive around honking their horns for everybody to see their artwork. There wasn't much snow on the streets, but every ounce of snow that fell in Lisbon that winter day was used for eating or making something artistic on top of car roofs that paraded down the streets. I can't even imagine enough snow to make everything outside white and so cold to the point of making the houses need heat inside.

Aunt Nelly's husband, who was a pharmacist also worked very hard, but when he got home she had dinner ready and the house was always beautiful and decorated with fresh flowers. Mercedes, her mother-in-law, had lived with them and had made her life pure hell. She'd died from colon cancer about eight years before Nelly's husband Ralph passed away also from cancer. The theory was that Mercedes had colon cancer because she ate hot peppers all the time and had burned her guts out. Nelly's husband tried everything he knew as a pharmacist to save his mother and besides giving her medicine he also gave her gold shots, which didn't save her but he believed did prolong his mother's life.

Nelly's husband made good money as a pharmacist, so she never had to work; she was a housewife and a mother and that was plenty of work. She never had maids, they are very expensive in North America, only rich people can afford one and they were not rich. Nelly did the family laundry and cooked and cleaned, that's why her arms were so big, from working so hard.

Mama and Aunt Heydee cried when they heard all of this and hugged their sister, feeling sorry for her because that was the kind of work that no woman should be subjected to unless she was a servant. Nelly was a young girl, a fragile flower when she had left Portugal.

She asked them not to feel sorry for her because she had been the happiest woman that ever existed and throughout her marriage each day was better than the day before.

Aunt Nelly had a vision when she landed at the Lisbon airport. She'd never had a vision in her life and she was embarrassed to tell her sisters. She was afraid that they might think she was crazy. After she descended the steps from the airplane, she saw her mother's ghost standing there and smiling at her the way she used to. She freaked out when she saw that. Mama told her that this meant that their mother had come to greet her and it only could be a good omen.

Weird, if I say so myself, I would not be happy to see a ghost, even if it was my grandmother smiling; I would be scared. Tomorrow morning Aunt Heydee is taking her sister Nelly to Paris for three days. I'll miss them both.

They are back! It was a bit disastrous between the two sisters. I heard Nelly tell Mama that Heydee was heartless. When they got to Paris, Nelly was feeling faint, and her heart was giving her trouble, and she didn't feel that she should go out that night. So, Aunt Heydee tucked her in bed at the hotel and said, "I am going to share my heart medicine with you. Here it is right next to you with a glass of water and the telephone number of a doctor, in case you get worse. I'll see you later."

I had to smile when I heard that. Aunt Heydee has never had a sick day in her life, and if she did, no one was aware of it because she never looks for sympathy. She is too busy to even bother with her own heart.

When Aunt Heydee heard Nelly complaining about being left alone to die in the hotel, she reasoned with Mama. "I am in Paris, and I'm going to stay in a hotel room holding her hand? Not me! The medicine was right there next to her, and as everyone can see she is still alive!"

I don't believe that Aunt Nelly will ever forgive Aunt Heydee.

"Poor Nelly," I heard Mama telling Aunt Heydee in the kitchen, "Imagine how she must have felt when his sperm fell inside her eye. Of course she cried scared, she thought she was going to go blind. He promised that he would never again ask her to do that. Her husband must have been a very understanding man; he loved her very deeply." They both agreed.

"Just the thought of it," said Aunt Heydee with a sigh, "What women have to go through to please their husbands." I wanted to ask them what sperm is but I have enough brains to realize that they would know that I was eavesdropping and would get yelled at. One thing was for sure; it has something to do with sex. My friend Julia from school told me that sperm is a men's form of menses and that's all she knows.

Nelly and I have good heart-to-heart talks. She told me she noticed I am treated like a child. She told me that in North America girls my age are treated like adults. She told me how much she misses her husband and how they used to take long walks every night after dinner and talk about all kind of subjects. He was a very intelligent man. They were both in love with each other, even after being married for so many years. Both her sons are very handsome and her daughter Ruth is also very beautiful, she is married and has a little girl whose name is Kim. Nelly feels lonely, and she would love to take me to North America with her. She told me she loves me and she gave me her picture as a memory to keep for myself. I put it in a small frame and I set it on my night table next to my bed.

Nelly shaves under her armpits! That is so American! She uses a dainty razor blade made for women. After using it a few times, she will throw the blade away, she told me. I have never seen such a thing. Papa has to make suds in a cup and uses a very sharp razor blade knife. He carefully stretches his skin between his fingers so he doesn't cut himself seriously, but he always nicks himself no matter how carefully he shaves his face. Once in awhile he goes to the barbershop and they put hot towels on his face like they do to all their clients to make the shaving smoother.

Nelly told me that all her clothes are bought in various department stores, where you can choose from hundreds of styles. Not here, I told her, we have to have a seamstress come to our house to make our dresses because the price tags in the clothing stores are very expensive and for tourists only. I do have fun looking through fashion magazines and picking the style of dress I would like to have, but it can't compare to going to a store and actually trying it on first before buying it. To top it off, the seamstress that comes to our house has horrible bad breath. While she is pinning the material on me I have to hold my breath the whole time. Mama knows about it, but she says beggars can't be choosers. Maria Josefina is the least expensive seamstress we know of and does a great job at sewing the dresses. Her price fits our budget.

Nelly has a movie camera and has been taking movies of all of us to take back to America. We went to the beach yesterday and she filmed Max-Leão showing his muscles as he lifted me up in the air. Max-Leão is into physical fitness and he works out lifting weights every day to build his muscles; he is very strong.

Nelly sure drinks a lot of soda. I don't like soda; it gives me bubbles in the stomach and then I feel bloated. She can drink the contents of a whole bottle of soda right from the bottle, all in one shot without taking a break to breathe, it's amazing! Must be the way Americans drink soda. We always put the soda inside of a glass and sip it little by little. If we are thirsty we drink water, but that's probably because we can't afford soda. Water is free.

Over the weekend, Nelly and I went on a mission trip. This is a secret between the two of us; she wanted to see if someone that she really liked when she was a younger girl is still alive. His name was Jorge João da Silva. According to her, he was the most handsome boy in the village where she had spent the last summer before going to North America. They were in love with each other but because he was Catholic the affair never went any further. She had thought about him many times through the years, and now that she was a widow she wanted to see him again.

251

So we took the train up north and went to the small village, Pedro da Cadeira. When we arrived, the people working at the train station knew exactly whom she was asking about. He was married and lived with his wife and family on a big farm on a hill. The train station manager offered to call him on the telephone and Aunt Nelly asked him to tell Jorge João da Silva he had a visitor from the past, but not to give her name. We waited at the train station and about half an hour later a man looking like an older John Wayne came walking our way. The meeting took my breath away. They looked at each other and they still recognized each other after thirty-four years. They ran towards each other, hugging each other as if the years had stood still. He took us to his house and introduced us to his wife who offered us lunch and seemed very happy to see us.

It was a wonderful day, and also a sad day because in my heart I was hoping that he was still single and they could have gotten married. I don't care if he is a Catholic or not, and I have a feeling that had Nelly found him a single man, she would have not cared about it either. Love would have conquered all. But at least now she knows that he is alive and happy.

Before getting on the train Nelly bought some very ripe and juicy plums, and we ate them on the train on our way back to Lisbon. When I got tired, she put my head on her shoulder and said, "Go ahead, little angel, take a little nap and rest." I love the way she talks to me.

Here it goes again, the *déjà vu* feeling. I was in my bedroom reading *The Count of Monte Cristo*, one of my very favorite books, except for *The Egyptian*, which is my number one favorite book to read over and over again, when Nelly came in and put on my bed the pictures of her two sons, Alberto and Joe. She asked me the same question Mama asked me a few years back, "Which one do you like the most?"

Hmm, I thought to myself, *doesn't she know that I am marrying Alberto? Why is she asking me this question?* I pointed to Alberto's picture without a word.

She smiled at me and said, "I was just making sure." I smiled back.

She is leaving tonight back to North America. I wish I could go with her.

My brothers and I were all in bed as we are supposed to be by nine o'clock, to get up early to go to school, when I heard Nelly asking, "Where's Verónica? I want to give her a kiss once again before leaving."

I heard Mama telling her, "She has school tomorrow, it's late, and she is already sleeping."

Nelly tiptoed into my bedroom and I made believe that I was sleeping, keeping my eyes closed. She bent forward and gave me a delicate kiss on my forehead. "Goodbye darling," she said, "I love you." And she left.

I cried and cried and asked God if there was one thing that I wished for with all my heart, it was to go to North America and live with Aunt Nelly, even if I had to sacrifice myself and marry her son. He can't be that bad since his mother is the most loving and caring person in the whole world. Then I thanked God for everything, like I try to do every night before sleeping.

I have a special prayer that I personally made up: Thank you God for everything you have given me. Please continue to protect us all, and bless our family, and João, from Costa da Caparica, whom I will never forget even though he was never my boyfriend; I still love him and wish him my very best.

Mama came to my bedroom a few days ago looking sad, and she pointed to Nelly's picture on the night-table next to my bed. "I can't help notice that you put her picture next to your bed and you don't have one of me, your own mother. I want you to know that she is not the nice person you think she is. She acted nice to you to cover her domineering personality. And besides that, she is also jealous of anyone that gets in her way." And Mama left my bedroom.

I opened the night-table top drawer and put Nelly's picture away. The only picture I have in my bedroom now is the one with my two young cousins who were taken to a concentration camp by the Nazis and killed in the gas chamber.

Mama dictated to me a letter in Spanish to send to my cousin Alberto, asking if Aunt Nelly had gotten home all right since it's been a week and we have not heard from her. I thought the whole idea was dumb and I didn't want to do it. "It's been only one week!" I argued back to Mama.

"So what?" She insisted, "You write exactly what I am going to dictate."

So I did, and in Spanish! My goodness, I don't like Spanish and don't understand Spanish.

Mama said the English I am learning in high school would not be enough to make me a writer, and Alberto doesn't understand Portuguese.

"Makes more sense that we write in Spanish," she said again. "Nelly lived with her mother-in-law who was from Morocco, and they only spoke Spanish at home. Therefore, Alberto most likely can read Spanish," she continued to reason, "If he doesn't understand Spanish, Nelly will translate for him."

Against my will I wrote in Spanish, "Dear Cousin Alberto, I am very worried. Something horrible must have happened to Aunt Nelly. I have not slept for the last three days concerned about her health. I know she has a bad heart, will you write to me at once with news of her condition?" I signed, "Your worried and distressed cousin Verónica."

I hate being manipulated by Mama to do things that I don't want to do.

A letter written in Spanish arrived the morning after I sent out Mama's letter to Cousin Alberto. Alberto had seen my pictures and home movies that Nelly had taken back with her to North America, and he would like me to write to him, because he liked me a lot. Obviously, the letter written by Mama in Spanish wondering about Nelly arriving safely had not arrived to North America yet.

Mama said we should wait for his next letter before I answered this one. Then Mama gave me a little piece of paper that she had kept hidden since I was born. Supposedly Alberto had written to me when he was twelve years old congratulating Mama on my birth, and on the other side of the small paper he had written in English, "I heard that you are a beautiful baby with green eyes and dark hair, will you marry me when you get older?"

His mother must have forced him to write such a note; no twelve-year-old boy would ask a baby girl to marry him. Just in case he did do that on his own, even though I doubt it, I put his note proposing marriage away in my jewelry music-box, as my first love letter ever received and read.

Another letter from North America arrived today. It was Alberto assuring me that Nelly was still living and doing well. Somehow I felt that he had written that letter with a touch of irony as if he was aware of the game being played. But then he went on again to say that he had seen my pictures and the film that his mother had taken home, and he had found me to be very pretty.

I was going to write back in my best English, but Mama said, no way, I was inept to do such a thing, she was going to coach me exactly on what words to write back.

Her writings are all poetic boring stuff that makes no sense. The only words that are mine are my signature. I feel so weird about this whole thing.

Summer of 1960

While on a trip to Belem, when nobody was watching, I carved on the trunk of a huge tree a little heart with the letters J and V, it stands for João and me in love forever. I no longer remember his face, but it feels right to have someone in my heart.

255

Letters come and go, all between Alberto and Mama. I write what she tells me to write in Spanish and then I sign it. I wonder if Nelly is also telling Alberto what to write, because in that case this love-letter exchange stuff is basically between Mama and her sister Nelly. I can't stand it. I want to believe it's him though; he has been sending me pictures of furniture and clothes all cut out from magazines.

He says he wants to know more about me. He wants to know what my favorite color is, and what do I like to do as a hobby. The answers are never mine, it's all answered like a mad poet in phrases that make no sense and don't even rhyme. I really don't know much about him except for a couple of pictures he sent me. And from me he is not getting any answer to his questions because Mama is on a mission of poetry in fantasyland, where reality is nonexistent.

Alberto has been sending me lots of pictures. My favorite one was taken ten years ago when he was in the United States Air Force and he is wearing his uniform. He was very handsome even though he is now older, twelve years older than I.

We are living in the country again for the summer. This is another forsaken place, away from civilization, with woods and lots of eucalyptus trees all around us. But somehow I like it better here than at Malveira. They don't pretend to be a town because there's nowhere to go. We have a huge forest behind our rental house that makes up for us being out nowhere and I spend the days lying in the hammock outside, reading my books in the shade of the trees. The next neighbor's farm is about a fifteen-minute walk, but we have no reason to meet them.

The letters continue to arrive from America, about one every two weeks. I am starting to get used to them, someone cares for me enough to bother to answer the dim-witted letters Mama writes. Maybe he likes the letters he is getting. What a horrible thought if he is not writing at all. In his last letter he asked me if I would consider being his girlfriend. Mama said yes, and wrote more Spanish love poetry back.

Aunt Heydee came by this weekend and took my brothers and me for a country hike. I love being with her; she is what life is all about. We walked and walked up the hill and then up a mountain, my very first real mountain hike. We got to the top and I made a wish to God, I want to climb mountains, tall ones and big wide ones, so that when I reach the top, I can see the earth all around me. I want to travel and see the world and have incredible adventures, and in every country that has a mountain, I will climb to the top.

Aunt Heydee knows all about the meaning of life, and as she stretched her arms out, she pointed to the land around and below us. "Take in the breath of life," she said for us all to hear, "Use your lungs and your eyes and all your senses, and live each day as a gift to be thankful for."

A few weeks ago Mama wanted to make sure that I was healthy. The result came back that I might have tuberculosis. They saw something on the film, and tomorrow I have to go back to the hospital and see Uncle Augusto for more lung X-rays.

Uncle Augusto didn't hug me. I was there alone in the big cold hospital building with no one to hold my hand. I felt very sad and lonely. If Aunt Heydee had not been in Venice for her vacation she would have been with me. They took a lot more X-rays, and Uncle Augusto had a concerned look on his face as he put his hand in front of him so that I would not come close to him. I must be dying, and worst of all I am contagious; he would not even give me a goodbye hug. He sent me back home, stating, "Tell your mother that I will call her later after I have some time to look at your lung X-rays."

Good news. I am fine. What they saw on the first X-ray was simply a scar that healed from when I had tuberculosis as a child. But, like Mama said, I am still not as strong as other

At the Top of the Mountain.

people, I will always be sickly and have to eat more than others, otherwise it could revert again into tuberculosis and I will die, just like our young maid Olivia who worked for us when I was just a baby.

Mama is always talking about her whenever the subject of tuberculosis comes up. Mama loved Olivia, who she considered a friend more than a maid. But Olivia was dying and used to cough a lot and spit blood. I probably caught tuberculosis from Olivia when I was a child.

Mama is on a mission of making me strong and healthy. She wakes me up in the middle of the night to give me pudding. I love pudding, but not in the middle of the night. She says she is sacrificing her own sleep by having to wake up to feed me, and the least I can do is be thankful. I have to eat every three hours a little something, as she says. She even bought me corn flakes so that I will drink milk with it. She loves me when I am sick. It pays to get sick, that's for sure. I love corn flakes with hot milk and lots of sugar on top of it. But pudding, even if it's chocolate pudding, in the middle of the night is more than I can stand.

Since the motorcycle accident Mama has developed a sixth sense. She is able to tell things that are going to happen in the future. She saved Max-Leão's life when she stopped him from going for a car ride with two other boys. His two friends got into a car accident and got killed. She also saved her brother Augusto's life by warning him not to go out on a certain day because something bad was going to happen. Besides poetry, she is now writing short stories too. Mama has also started painting, which is really strange since before the accident she couldn't even help me draw a vase. Now she is doing all kinds of paintings with oil on canvas.

I am doing well; basically healthy if it wasn't for the sharp knife like pains I have on and off in my legs. Like Uncle Augusto says, I have rheumatoid arthritis and I have to learn to live with it. There isn't much that can be done except rubbing my legs, taking sour medicine, and sitting outside in the sun. Nothing really helps.

Mama gave Max-Leão and I some money for the two of us to take a bus to Eiriceira. She had to go to Lisbon to have José treated for asthma. The experimental drugs they are giving him now make him act weird and they are not helping him with the asthma.

Max-Leão and I decided to hitchhike to Eiriceira and save the bus money to buy goodies when we got there. It took us over an hour standing on the road with our thumbs up. The young couple that picked us up told us we were foolish to travel this way because there were people out there picking up children to hurt them. We know all that, but it's not going to happen to us, we are very careful; besides, we already had plans to take the bus home before it gets dark.

It was a wonderful day at the beach. We bought a nice-sized watermelon from a street vendor and we climbed the rocks with it and the lunch box we had brought with us. We set up our stuff and clothes safely under the shade of one of the rocks, and ran right into the water where we stayed for hours until we had purple lips and were shaking cold.

Both seated on the rock cliff, we had our codfish-cakes and bread. We didn't bring any utensils to eat with because it was all finger food, so we didn't have a knife to cut the watermelon. The solution was simple; Max-Leão picked the watermelon up in the air and then splashed it into one pointy rock, splitting the watermelon into pieces. We used our tongues and teeth and hands and we ate until our stomachs were bloated. We sat drenched in watermelon juice on the seashore under the warm sunrays, watching the waves coming up towards us.

When we got home, we told Marcia our maid, about our adventure and she told us there was a party going on at the next farm with people our own age and we should go and have fun. We washed up quickly and took a walk to the neighbor's farm.

Cool Watermelon on a Summer Day.

It was a hot summer night, and everyone outside on the wide marble veranda was dancing or talking in groups. The lady of the house introduced me to a few boys and girls my own age and we were there about ten minutes, talking, when Inácio, one of the boys in the group, asked me to dance. He was just putting his arm around my waist when Marcia showed up all flustered and nervous.

"Let's go," she said, grabbing my arm and pulling me away from my dancing partner. I was so embarrassed, feeling like a baby being taken home by the maid. I mumbled an excuse to Inácio.

Mama had come back from her trip to Lisbon and had found out from Marcia that Max-Leão and I had hitchhiked that day and were now at a party.

She was not happy.

As always, I got blamed for it, and she said as punishment I was not allowed to return to the party because I was the eldest, and should have had more brains than to hitchhike with Max-Leão.

Marcia felt really bad but what she doesn't realize is that Mama would have found any excuse to get us both out of the party where Max-Leão and I would be among people our own age. We were allowed to have dinner before we were sent to bed, but I wasn't hungry.

"*Psst, psst,*" I heard Papa calling me this morning as I was going across the hallway. He was sitting alone at the dining room table and had just finished his usual cup of coffee, one soft-boiled egg, and two pieces of toast with butter, for breakfast. "Verónica," he whispered, as if worried Mama might hear him, "sit down next to me, and listen to me. I want you to know that what your mother is doing, you know — setting you up for a marriage with your cousin — someone that you don't even know, is wrong in my opinion. She believes it is the best for you, but as your father I have doubts. What do you think?"

Caught by surprise and being pushed into thinking about a situation that I didn't want to face wasn't easy.

"I don't mind," I answered him, barely speaking up, and I mumbled, "It's okay with me." And I looked away as if afraid that he could read my fears.

"Be careful, daughter," he said, "you just turned sixteen years old, you are still a child in my opinion. Make sure you love this person before you marry him. Marriage is a lifetime commitment. If you change your mind; I am on your side."

I didn't know what to say except, "Okay, thanks, Papa." And I left the room.

Papa rarely talks to me; his concern took me by surprise. I was speechless, but what could I say? Have a heart-to-heart talk with a man that I am afraid to talk back to and don't even know, except that he is my father and he intimidates me most of the time. I had to smile though when I left the room, for Papa does care for me, and he is worried.

There's no going back. My future is somewhere else. Like the gipsy woman foretold already, each of Mama's children are like stars, each is destined to go a different direction. My destiny is going to North America and being happy.

The turkey was served for dinner, but no one was able to eat a bite. We just stared at it and ate the potatoes and the vegetables instead. Since we arrived here last month this turkey had taken a liking to Mama. The other chickens, ducks, and turkeys went on with their normal daily business; but this one loved "Mama Linda." Since the accident Papa calls Mama, "Linda." She likes the new name, and we all make her happy by calling her Mama Linda, principally if we are trying to get on her good side.

When she walked in the garden the turkey would run towards her and then walk along her like a pet dog on a leash, and when she would sit down he would lie down by her feet. One morning her bedroom window was opened and the turkey jumped on her windowsill and just stood there, staring at her. That really freaked her out and she no longer thought it was funny. After that incident our maid felt that the turkey was possessed by some lost soul.

The Turkey and Mama.

Aunt Heydee came all the way from Lisbon just to meet the turkey. After all, turkeys are stupid and have no feelings, just like the chickens and other animals that we eat, and that's why they get eaten; they are not smart enough to run away and hide. Uncle Augusto and his family paid us a visit too. Everybody wanted to see the possessed turkey. But the maid got Mama all flustered, and between her and the neighbors coming by they got Mama to believe that killing the turkey would set the soul free.

So it was done, killing the turkey was for the best, they all agreed, but when it came time to eat the bird, one had to wonder if the soul was still inside, and nobody was going to take that chance.

Aunt Heydee is so smart; besides Portuguese of course she speaks fluent French, Italian, Spanish, and English. She is a woman of the world, seen everything and done everything except being married. She won't budge on her requirements for the perfect husband, and she will not settle for anything less than what she feels she deserves. He must be Jewish, otherwise the family would dishonor her; rich, because she has been poor long enough; educated, because she needs someone that she can talk to on her intellectual level; a lot younger than her, so that he can keep up with her active lifestyle; and handsome, because getting married will be enough of a sacrifice for her, and the truth is that she would like someone that is pleasant to look at. Sensitive and loving is a must, yet he has to be masculine with lots of muscles like Hercules. He must own his own private home in the city for the winter months as well as a villa in the country for the summer months, and— at top of the list — he must love opera.

She has told me about her travels through other countries of Europe, from the caverns on the Island of Capri to the Swiss Alps, from Rome's Coliseum to Paris' catacombs, and even though she travels by herself she has no problems making friends along the way. Every day is an awesome day of adventure and wonder. She is a self-taught French and piano teacher, and she dabbles successfully in oil painting. She never went past fourth grade, yet she is a self-made master of everything she does.

Yesterday, while we were seated on the hammock outside, she told me how much she appreciates beauty as well as what someone else might consider to be ugly. Everything has a place in the palette of Mother Nature, she said. As an artist, she sees men and women as an incredible creation, and through her drawings and oil paintings she has grown to appreciate all forms and shapes.

"There is nothing ugly in the world," she told me, "it's all perception, how you look at it. Life is very much like a diamond and it shines as long as you keep it polished."

She always gives thanks to God for being able to see, feel, and touch.

When I return to Lisbon, Aunt Heydee is going to start taking me along with her on her weekend adventures, and Mama said it was okay. I need culture in order to make a good impression on Alberto; otherwise he's going to send me back to Portugal.

Aunt Ligia came into my bedroom before we left Lisbon to spend our summer in the country and she tried to make conversation with me about different topics that in her opinion are essential between a man and a woman for a happy marriage.

I didn't respond well to her interview. Matter of a fact, I failed miserably because I didn't feel like I had much to say about anything, so I didn't. Aunt Ligia and I have never been in a close relationship; she is too nervous for me. Besides that, she accused me, a few years ago when I started writing children's stories, of plagiarizing the children's stories she wrote and used to read to me when I was a child. I don't have any recollection of that happening; I must have been a baby. Anyway, she reported to Mama that I was completely without graces and my culture was equal to a rusty nail found deep in mud. I had nothing to offer a cultured man like Alberto, an American and an engineer. Aunt Ligia told

Mama that she'd better do something drastic about my personality, which amounts to a flat expression of nodding, staring, and "yes" or "no" answers. In other words, I am boring. I knew that.

Autumn of 1960

We all said goodbye to Max-Leão last week. He was sent to England to become an architect. Mama cries a lot. I don't cry about it but I miss him. Papa's family are paying for Max-Leão's upkeep and overseeing his education in London. Mama says that a mother has to make sacrifices like this for the welfare of her child, and for the same reason she will be sending me away to North America as soon as Alberto asks for my hand in marriage.

Personally, I feel like Mama is trying to get rid of all of us and I feel confused about my situation.

It's not the same without Max-Leão. I do not see eye-to-eye with José. Basically we stay away from each other because we don't have anything in common. Mama sent us out to the movies a couple of times, and he always disappears around a street corner, getting lost within the crowd. I feel so stupid and abandoned when he does that, so I refuse to go out with him. Last week when we went through the busy street of Madalena, which is known for crime and prostitution, he took a quick turn around the street corner and once again disappeared out of my sight. He does that all the time. I went to the movies by myself.

I told Mama about it and he was excused as being too young and just a boy. He is spoiled and gets away with everything he does. He is supposed to let us know when he leaves the house, but he just opens the front door and yells goodbye as he slams the door behind him. He gives us no time to ask him where he is going. He is also very good at making money deals at school; because our *escudos* have certain small size coins that have more value than larger size ones. He has convinced some students to trade their small coins for his larger ones. So he gets into trouble at school. But Mama says that if the kids in his class fall for the size of the coin instead of its value, then they deserve to be cheated out of their money.

The other day José made me angry, and I told him that I would never ask him to come and live with me in North America because he is a crook and a liar and he will be put in jail and then he will be going to the electric chair to pay for his crimes. I know it was mean for me to do that, but he is constantly irritating me. He is a pest!

I have thought a few times in the past, and still in the present, that if I could find a way to leave this world I would do it. I don't like anything about my life, but I am too much of a coward to take a chance at hurting myself. Poison can't be pleasant. I read the book *Madame Bovary* and I didn't think it was romantic when she killed herself the way she did. I can't even imagine more stomach cramps than when I have my monthly period. I thought about jumping from a bridge, but it has to hurt like hell when you hit the hard ground even if it's just for a few minutes. Jumping from a bridge into the river Tejo, was another thought, but since I can't swim, I'd be swallowing water like the victims of the Inquisition when they had water forced down their throat until they died — and that has to be as nasty as that time when I was a kid and that beach boy dunked me under the ocean, not a very pleasant experience. I could try what Max-Leão did with his chemistry experiment in the bathroom, but I would have to make sure that no holes were left for the gas to escape, and with my luck I'd be discovered and beaten to a pulp.

My future is locked with my Aunt Nelly and Cousin Alberto in North America. They are the only ones who can help me, and I know because I tried to run away to Spain a few days ago and it was an eye-opening experience.

I went to a traveling agency and the price of a train ticket is more than ten years of my allowance, not to mention I would need money to buy food and rent an apartment while waiting to get a job. I am only sixteen years old and no one is going to hire someone my age. I don't have any skills except for stuffing envelopes or writing addresses like I do at Papa's office, I don't know anything else. School has not taught me anything that I can use in the outside world. I can't even be a bum living in the streets of Spain because, when other bums would speak to me, I wouldn't even know what they were saying as I don't understand a word of Spanish.

I was walking home from the American Embassy where I have been spending a few hours in the afternoon listening to musical records and reading books, and a boy on the street saw me and followed me home. Then, about seven o'clock, I heard the sound of a guitar and someone singing a love song. I looked out of my window and there he was, with a friend playing a guitar across the street and facing our building. I went out into the veranda of my bedroom and smiled happily. He took a courtesy bow acknowledging my presence and threw me a kiss with his hand as he started to sing, "Your green eyes are like the sea, tell me that you are the one for me. I love you, I love you, let me kiss your sweet lips and show my love for you."

Josefina the maid was the only one home besides me, and said, "I'll take care of them, just watch, Miss Verónica." And she took off from the veranda and out of my room.

I had no idea what she was going to do. I was standing at the veranda enjoying his singing until I saw Josefina return from the kitchen with a pail of water. She stepped onto the veranda and asked them with a big smile if they could get a little closer to the building so that we could hear them better. When they promptly followed her invitation, she lifted the bucket of cold water and dropped the whole thing on the two boys. They took off, cursing at both of us. I will never know who my Romeo was. I doubt he will ever return to serenade under my bedroom window.

A package from North America arrived today. It is a silver engagement ring with six brilliant stones all around. Alberto had enclosed a little note with it. "Verónica, will you be my fiancé?"

Mama wrote back saying, "Yes."

Now that I am engaged and have a real boyfriend I can show my ring to everyone in school.

My friends at school were shocked by the news of my engagement. Laura, who walks home with me, showed a lot of concern and offered me her house if I wanted to hide away. She told me that I was nuts to go along with this charade. What if Alberto gets here and he doesn't look like his picture? He may be missing his legs or be blind or be very old or be plain nasty, smelly and ugly, she told me. I assured her that he was on the level because his mother is my mother's sister and she is a wonderful lady. Besides, I am in love with him and I am not afraid, I told her defiantly.

"I will get engaged too, then," said Laura, getting upset over the whole thing as if this was some kind of a contest between the two of us, "I am not going to let you go ahead of me and get married, I am not going to be an old maid."

I told Mama about what Laura had said, and Mama told me that Laura was not to be trusted anymore as a friend, she was obviously jealous, and that's why she said stuff like that.

As soon as I got into school today, Laura grabbed me in the hallway to show me her diamond engagement ring. I didn't even know that she had a boyfriend. She couldn't wait to show it to me. She is engaged and will be married when she turns eighteen years old. I am very happy for her.

Mama has told me that I will not be returning to high school in January. There's no need to learn anymore school stuff. What I need is a different type of education, the kind that will prepare me for being a wife. She signed me up to start this January at a school that will teach me proper manners and how to cook French-style and sew pretty dresses for myself. As of January it is official: Aunt Heydee is in charge of the cultural part of my education.

I said goodbye to everybody in school. From now on I will be busy spending time with Aunt Heydee and getting ready for the future, which does not include anyone here. I am better off breaking my roots now and not holding on to anything or anybody. Encarnação is my friend, but she has her family and can't leave Portugal. Aunt Heydee is in the same predicament; she says North America is for the young people like me. Max-Leão is gone and José is just someone that lives here. I am alone. But I long for love, whatever that is that everyone speaks and writes about all the time. Love is in songs and books, and it's understood that once you find it you will always be happy. I would like to be happy.

Winter of 1961

Aunt Heydee goes out every night to dance or hang out with her girlfriends at the coffee shops, but she doesn't suffer from getting into a cold bed when she comes home. The maid gets 50 *centavos* to sleep in Aunt Heydee's bed until she gets home, then the maid goes to her bedroom and Aunt Heydee gets to sleep in the warmed bed. Her bed is next to mine and I watch her as she sleeps with a bunch of pillows so that her head is kept up and her face doesn't get squished down. She doesn't have a single line in her face; she attributes it to sleeping almost sitting and of course using almond oil on her skin everyday. It works!

Alberto has sent me a home movie and more pictures so that I can get to know him better. There's a lot of snow where he lives. I can't wait to play in the snow and throw snowballs at him and make a huge snowman. When I go to North America I am going to have lots of bubble baths like Doris Day, and wear clothes bought in a store, and have lots of ice cream whenever I want, and sing and dance every day with loud American rock and roll music.

Things in Africa are pretty scary and getting worse as more and more of our colonies are becoming independent from Portugal. There are lots of ill feelings as the African people are trying to get the white people out. Horrible atrocities are committed everyday. The newspapers tell stories of crimes against white women and children who are in the way of black people becoming independent from Portuguese control. It's an ugly, nasty time in history, and innocent people get caught in between the ignorance and savage behavior of everyone on both sides. I hope and pray that Amelia and her family are safe living in Africa.

The *Diário de Notícias* blurted out an episode of utter horror; when an eleven-year-old black boy was walking in one of the streets of Lisbon some men from a garage grabbed him as if he was a criminal from Africa. They got the gasoline hose and used it as an enema; they killed the little black boy. I cried before I went to sleep. I felt that I could also be a criminal very easily. If I had a chance to do it, I would have killed those men that tortured the little boy. I would like to kill them with my own hands, those bastards! From now on I will never read the news.

In order for me to leave Portugal right after the wedding, all the paperwork with the civil wedding has to be arranged ahead of time. The Portuguese and the American Embassy are working together, but very slowly. If I am to leave with Alberto to North America, I have to marry him by proxy as soon as possible, and that means I will have to marry Uncle Augusto, who will represent Alberto here in Portugal. Because Uncle Augusto is a medical doctor, he has a lot of influence with the government and the needed paperwork can get speed up, otherwise it could take years for me to be approved to leave. Being married to an American will also expedite the procedure. When Alberto comes to Portugal to pick me up, I will already be married to him legally. Alberto only has one week off from work, so everything has to be ready for the real wedding within a few days after he arrives, and hopefully we will be married religiously after three days so that we can have three days of honeymoon before leaving Portugal. I am nervous but not scared. I am enjoying the attention that everybody gives me, and wondering what other wonderful things are ahead in my life.

The civil wedding went very well, even though the "real" groom was missing. Everybody got dressed up, and Augusto's wife Coty was there smiling at the whole event and so were their youngest daughter Rica Gilda, Aunt Heydee, and Aunt Gimol, who is Grandma Rica's youngest sister. It felt like a real wedding with guests, flowers, and signatures.

Papa never smiled throughout the wedding and Mama was very fidgety. I felt she was scared I would back out of this compromise. She doesn't realize that I will do anything to get out of here and go live with Aunt Nelly. I wore one of the dresses Alberto had sent me and I held a bouquet of flowers just like a bride would. Pictures were taken inside the courthouse and outside, and while we were out there posing for the photographer a woman going by said out loud to her friend, "Foolish girl — obviously she is marrying the old goat, for his money!"

We all laughed, having a good time. Aunt Coty was hysterical and laughed the loudest. The woman passerby probably thought that we were all bizarre.

It's opera season with Aunt Heydee. No wonder she is called "Napoleão #1:" She took me to the famous São Carlos Opera House and she introduced herself as a journalist and me as her assistant. This is the way we get into the *hot spots* of culture without paying. I am not to tell Mama, as she would not approve. Aunt Heydee cannot afford a ticket at São Carlos; she has a meager salary as a private French teacher and she saves every penny she earns to go on vacation during

Marrying Uncle Augusto.

the summer months. Her food is carefully planned daily, healthy but small meals. Her clothes are handmade from other people's hand-me-downs. She is a survivor in a tough world. She is a woman without a man to support her and take care of her. As she has told me so many times, "You either grab life by the horns, or you lie down and die. The choice is yours."

Things didn't go as we planned. Aunt Heydee and I got separated inside the famous glittery São Carlos Theatre. It was the opening night of a Portuguese opera, which meant over crowding. Aunt Heydee was pushed along with the crowd to the seats below and I was sent upstairs with an usher. Don't know for sure how it happened, but the usher took me to a private balcony, a few spaces from the presidential compartment. I could tell because it was centrally located and had the Portuguese flag draped in front of it.

Meagerly dressed in my Scottish-pattern brown flannel dress, I sunk myself into the red velvet seat so I would not be seen, then carefully I took a peek out of my balcony, trying to see where Aunt Heydee was seated downstairs.

I was afraid that someone would come upstairs, grab me by the hair, and throw me out of the theatre. It was obvious I didn't belong in this sophisticated gathering of men in tuxedos and women all glittered up with long beautiful dresses. Everybody was dressed for the opera except me.

The São Carlos is the most famous opera theatre in Lisbon, and probably the most famous in all of Portugal. It is a magnificent theatre with gold encrusted balconies and huge chandeliers hanging from its painted ceilings, which depicts what seems to be famous opera scenes. Only rich people that love opera can afford the expensive tickets. I saw Aunt Heydee down below; she smiled at me and waved. I waved back. During intermission I intended to run downstairs and join her. I was proud of myself being so close to the president's balcony, even though it looked like he wasn't going to attend, since it was empty.

The lights went out, the door behind me opened, and three boys about my age came in. They were as surprised as I was. One of them sat next to me, introducing himself as the son of some guy I'd never heard of, as if that was going to impress me. The opera had started. I moved my chair away from his, but he moved his chair next to me, making sure his knee was touching mine. I kept moving until I was cornered into the wall. One of his friends said, "Why don't you leave the girl alone?" But he would not listen. He tried to make conversation and wanted to know if I had a boyfriend.

I said yes, and I was getting married officially in May of next year.

He went on to talk about how one year was too long to wait and a kiss from me would not hurt anybody.

What a retard! My luck, I always get stuck with jerks.

Then he put his arm over my shoulder, saying, "Give me a kiss."

I pushed him away. "No, I don't want to kiss you."

He was not giving up that easy. "And why not?"

I didn't know what to say, so I figured that if I shocked him he might leave me alone. With a very dignified look I said, "Because I don't know you, and I am Jewish!" I am such an idiot, but what else could I say?

After being taken aback for a bit, he remarked, "I don't care what you are, I will kiss you even if you are Jewish."

I pushed him away again the best I could, since I was so nervous I thought I was going to cry, and said, "I am not allowed to kiss someone that's not Jewish; it's against my religion." He came closer to my face and I pushed him away with my hand once again.

He finally got upset and said, "Well, Miss Jewish Special, if that's the way you feel." And he moved away.

Lucky for him, because I was starting to consider the idea that I might have to punch him if necessary. I was embarrassed and a nervous wreck. I have to admit that he was very cute, but he was definitely a "teddy boy," the latest from England to describe an immature bratty young villain.

The São Carlos Opera House.

The opera was boring and silly with a bunch of people screaming to the sound of a full orchestra, as if that could help the singers. Opera singing doesn't sound as natural and soul- moving like rock and roll. I found out that night, that nothing is worse to my ears than Portuguese opera. Opera is bad enough in a foreign language, but in Portuguese it's even more annoying than Italian. I hate opera. Intermission came and I ran out of the compartment and down the wide luxurious golden-carpeted steps.

I took a deep breath of relief when I saw Aunt Heydee in the foyer. We both sat together downstairs for the second part of the show. People seemed to have left for good during intermission because now there were plenty of seats available downstairs.

"I almost fainted when I saw you up there with three boys, are you all right?" she asked.

Still trembling from the experience I had gone through I said, yes, I was fine.

She encouraged me to keep this whole thing between the two of us. Mama would have her head if she found out about this incident.

~ *Chapter Seven* ~

Engaged to Cousin Alberto

1961

Spring of 1961

The school I am attending now is definitely a bride's school. The girls seem older than me, and have a lot more experience about life. I just sit through the sewing classes and manners classes and cooking classes. The students have their own little clique, and I don't dare tell anyone that I am already married to my cousin from America who I never met. I know I am not the smartest person, but I know enough not to say anything and be ridiculed. They call me an existentialist. When I was in high school I was called that too I take it as a compliment and an achievement, because everybody else is like a cookie cutter copy of each other, I can be myself and I don't have to explain why. I like being an existentialist.

I have seen movies with existentialists like me. They live in cities like New York and Paris too. They go out at night dressed in black to dark smoky nightclubs. Their hair is straight and they don't wear makeup. They are natural and love natural things. They are in touch with the Earth and do meditation. They dance to jazz and try to understand the meaning of life. They are unhappy, like me.

I love using the school's modern bathroom because they have perfumed hand soap. I lock the door and start by washing my feet first in the sink. All those years of ballet have paid off; I have no problem reaching the sink with my feet. After my feet, I wash my armpits. We don't have soft perfumed soap at home. I feel sparkly clean when I leave their bathroom. Sometimes someone will ask me what's taking me so long in there. I always say the same, "upset stomach."

The girls in this school are always acting like grownups and talking about world stuff. The other day between classes we were waiting in the hallway for the next class and they were talking about the Russian army and what would happen if they attacked Portugal. Some said they would rather kill themselves than submit to some fat Russian, others were saying to act nice towards them and they wouldn't kill you after they rape you.

I have to smile about all this because by the time the Russians get here to rape them, I will be in North America.

It's so much fun receiving presents from Alberto. I anxiously visit the mailbox every morning. When I don't get a letter I feel disappointed. I love the cards he sends me. My favorite card is the one where a red paper heart pops out on a spring. He wrote, "In America, today is Valentine's Day, and you are my sweetheart." I like that name sweetheart. *Sweet* is sugar; *heart* is love, *sweetheart* is such a perfect word. Americans are so smart with their language and expressions of love.

Every day I wear the earrings that Nelly gave me when she was here visiting us. They are the only earrings I wear.

Alberto is spoiling me with gifts, this week I got a box with two more dresses, summer cotton dresses; the seamstress comes over and fixes them to fit me better. I like Alberto's taste in clothing, simple and comfortable styles. He also sends me cutouts from magazines with the latest American styles of furniture. He wants me to pick the ones I like and send the pictures back, this way he learns more about my taste in furniture. I have fun marking a little cross on the pictures I like, and then Mama has me writing back to Alberto in her poetic Spanish madness.

Mama continues to dream of becoming a millionaire, and she is sure any day now she will win the million *escudos* lottery. I don't believe in that stuff. She has been playing for years the same lottery number her father used to buy when he was alive. Every week she buys a lottery ticket. Even when we were poor she always bought a ticket. She thinks that the day she doesn't buy it, that's going to be the week she will lose the big one. Sometimes she wins a few *escudos* and that convinces her even more that she is due to win the real thing any time soon. In my opinion, she is wasting her money on a lost cause. When she is not feeling well enough to go out, she asks me to go all the way downtown just to buy a lottery ticket from a specific guy who sells the tickets on a specific street corner.

I always tell her, "You are wasting your money, Mama, and you are not going to win."

She gets upset and tells me I just took her lucky chance away by blurting out a bad omen.

"Okay," I tell her, "Don't get the ticket, then."

And she says, "No, I'll take a chance anyway, even though you bring me bad luck. Go, get the ticket and think positive thoughts about it."

It would be nice if she won the lottery, but I really don't believe that she ever will.

For my birthday I got a funny greeting card from Alberto. A little bunny popped with stretched arms and it said on the bottom, "I love you this much." A little package arrived the next morning. Inside there was a gold bracelet with hearts all around. This is a love present and I like staring at it and feeling the little hearts in my hands. I wonder if he really loves me. He must, otherwise he would not be sending me such expensive gifts.

When I go out, I make sure my left hand is in view for everyone to see. The love bracelet and the ring state that I will soon be married. Lots of work is ahead to make sure that all the papers are in order so that I can leave for America with him next year. Aunt Nelly will be coming with Alberto for the wedding. They are bringing the wedding gown I chose from a magazine he sent me.

Summer of 1961

Since Mama was away with Papa for a weekend in Spain, I felt it was a good idea if I answered the letter I received from Alberto this morning. I wrote in English, "Dear Alberto, I love you too and I can't wait to see you in May, love and kisses, Verónica."

When Mama came back from her trip she was concerned that I might have spoiled everything with some silly girly stuff, and Alberto was going to change his mind about marrying me. In her opinion I should have waited for her to come back from Spain.

Alberto wrote back saying that he was thrilled I had finally written in English and he would be a lot happier if I could continue to write in English. Mama immediately made me write that I was terrible at writing in English, and I promised that from now on I would continue to write my feelings of love towards him in Spanish.

Mama gets a real kick out of Alberto calling her Brigitte Bardot. He always writes at the end of each letter, "Give B.B. a kiss from me." Mama doesn't look anything like B.B. I believe he is very diplomatic and he is trying to be friendly with his Aunt and future mother-in-law.

Mama came into my bedroom last night saying that we needed to talk. She stood by the dresser looking down at me while I stayed seated on my bed.

"You must not let anything silly, like thinking you are beautiful, get into your head. You are an average girl. At your age I was a real vamp." She took a long breath and continued, "One young man died because he knew I could never be his, so he killed himself. All my sisters were pretty, but I was a real knockout."

I stared at her, nodding my head in agreement as I was wondering why she constantly makes me feel like a worthless nobody, and what was she trying to tell me?

She finished, saying, "Remember, you are a plain girl, nothing special. You must accept that, or you will be very unhappy." Then she left the bedroom.

I don't know what got into her. Maybe she saw me pose in front of the mirror in my bedroom before I go to bed. I like to pose in front of the mirror and dance and smile and act like an actress. I always brush my hair before going to bed. One hundred strokes is the requirement for shiny healthy hair, but I never count. I don't feel unattractive, and I truly believe that I am pleasant to look at. Maybe she is afraid that I am getting vain, or maybe Aunt Heydee told her about the man we met in the trolley a few days ago. He came up to her and introduced himself as a movie agent as he handed her a calling card, saying very politely, "I couldn't help but notice your daughter. She is very attractive. Please consider bringing her to my studio, just call my office for an appointment." He left the trolley at the next stop.

Mama never tells me anything straight; she always has to beat around the bush. This is why I have not told anyone about the two sailors that stopped in front of me as I walked past them in downtown Lisbon a few days ago. One said to the other, pointing at me, "My goodness, what an incredible creation, and to think that this girl is the product of her parents fucking in the dark."

This was the worst language I had ever heard, but as I kept walking away from them, I couldn't help but smile as I

283

realized immediately that from the sailors' blunt point of view, they had paid me a great compliment.

It's been a lonely month. Aunt Heydee is somewhere in Morocco doing her once-a-year, one-month vacation. It's hot and lonely in the city. We are not going away this year; we are spending the summer in Lisbon. I fill my days by taking a daily bus ride to the airport to stand by the fence watching the planes coming and going. Other times, I take the ferryboat across the River Tejo. I don't look or talk to anyone. I just look at the world as if I was the only one, and I welcome its arms around me, protecting me from anyone that might want to hurt me. I get off the ferryboat, look around as if I am meeting someone, and then take the ferryboat back.

Mama doesn't have to worry about me going anywhere by myself. I have been taught well. I don't trust anybody and I have gotten used to staying within my own boundaries. I am faceless. No one can tell if I am sad or happy. Feeling this way keeps me protected from the outside, dormant until I wake up. Soon I'll be married and happy.

When a neighbor asked Mama, "How can you let Verónica, your only daughter, go to North America. It's too far away. Most likely you won't see her again. Aren't you going to miss her?"

She responded in the same manner as she did when she sent Max-Leão to England: "As a mother I must make sacrifices. I'd rather have my daughter far away and happily married than close by and without a future."

Everybody admires her utter sacrifice, and she is very self-righteous about that. She will not stop me from being happy even if she doesn't see me anymore. I can't wait to leave.

I saw a black person this afternoon, but it wasn't a good experience. I have learned there's good and bad in people of all races. I was walking a few blocks from home and my

By the Fence at the Airport.

right hand hit somebody between the legs, that's how close this black man was walking next to me. I said, "Excuse me," and I kept walking, but soon realized that he was doing that on purpose and once again my hand touched his leg, so I stopped and he stopped and smiled at me. I started walking faster and he started walking faster along with me, as if glued to my side. I thought about using my safety pin, but he was too big and it would probably feel like the bite of an ant on his leg.

He must have seen my angry face, because as I ran the rest of the way home he didn't follow me. I feel sad that some black people are as bad as white folks. I didn't tell anyone about what happened.

Autumn of 1961

Aunt Heydee is back. Thank God! I went out a few times with Aunt Morena last month, but I was embarrassed to be with her. She purposely pulls her skirt up as far as she can to show her legs while making "google eyes" and smiling to any man sitting across from her in the bus or the trolley. It doesn't even bother her that she doesn't know them. She winks at men when they walk past her on the street, it doesn't even matter what they look like. She acts like a loose woman and I can't help feeling ashamed to be with her.

Aunt Morena has told me stories about her dating experiences. She met a man at a dancing hall and he asked her to go with him to his car. She did, because she thought he wanted to be with her to talk and get to know each other better, but when he tried to take her clothes off she fought him and he got angry and beat her. The police were called upon the scene when people going by heard her screaming. She told me that she has to have a man in her life. She sure gets into a lot of trouble looking for love. In my opinion she is too desperate.

This summer Papa almost fired Aunt Morena because of what she did in his office. But Mama convinced Papa that all he had to do was move Morena's desk away from the window. Supposedly, while she was seated at her desk, she was lifting her skirt even further up than she does while riding the city's public transportation. With her legs open, she was trying to entice the man across the street, living in the third floor apartment across from Papa's office. This was going on for a while until the man's wife started to wonder why her husband would come home from work and go straight to their balcony window. That's when she caught her husband red-handed staring at Aunt Morena's crotch.

Aunt Morena's alibi was simple, she was very hot and the only way to cool off was to take her panties off and open her legs. It wasn't her fault that the neighbor was a peeping tom. She has told me several times that after twelve years of waiting patiently for a divorce from her womanizing, alcoholic husband, she is very lonely.

The "night man" as we all call him, is like the invisible man, and I wonder sometimes if he is from this planet. You don't see him while walking the streets, but you know he is there, like a salamander blended into the city walls. When Aunt Heydee forgets the key for the front door downstairs she does her usual thing, she claps her hands a few times, and there, right out of the shadows, is the "night man" with all the keys of the block.

He hardly says much, "Good evening ladies, forget the keys again, *hmm*?" And he opens the door for us after Aunt Heydee gives him 25 *centavos*.

It's freaky to say the least; I mean, what kind of a job is that, hiding in the night shadows waiting for someone to clap their hands to get help opening the front door. Freaky, freaky! And who is paying him I should ask, he couldn't be living from the 25 *centavos* that Aunt Heydee gives him whenever she forgets her house keys.

Mama told me that I am not to go out with Aunt Morena ever again. She has been officially banned from our home. She was caught stealing money from Papa's office. She had been stealing since Papa hired her two years ago to do office work. Papa only hired her as a favor because she is Mama's sister and needed a job. She is not being sent to prison, because she promised she would pay the monies she owes to Papa's company. The money was supposed to be going to artists without hands or arms that paint with their mouth or their feet and depend solely on the profit of selling their cards and calendars to make a decent living. This incident has put much shame on our family, and the name Morena is not spoken in our house. Papa will be putting the stolen monies into the company out of his own pocket, and Aunt Morena has promised to pay him monthly payments until it's all paid for.

Mama has cried a lot about this whole affair. Aunt Morena is not only man-hungry; she is not to be trusted. She steals from her own family, just like her perverted son Leão, whom I saw, a few years ago when I was a kid, stealing a silver ashtray from one of our cousins' houses when we were visiting them.

Mama told us that after Aunt Morena pays Papa what she owes him; she will open our home to her sister again. Aunt Morena may be wicked, but she is still her sister. Having the name Morena, meaning "tan" or "dark," must have been hard to live with, while my mother was called Branca, "white" like Snow White.

Names like Morena have an innuendo of negativity which can dictate someone's general characteristics as they grow up, said Papa.

I understand what he means to say, because my name is Verónica, which will always be associated with Saint Verónica, so I can never be a bad person, at least not with a clear conscience.

Mama told Papa how, as children, Morena was always treated as the black sheep of the family, no pun intended. She had grown used to being called "dark," and everybody had agreed that the name fit her since she had darker skin and was the ugly duckling. She never finished second grade. They treated her like a maid, sending her out to do errands for everybody. She had grown in the streets, being smart and corrupted by the people she hung out with. When she married a man who was not Jewish, that marked her even more as an outcast. When she moved with her husband to the island of Azores, everyone quietly agreed the farther the better. After Mama told this story, Papa felt sorry for Aunt Morena and said, "If you call a child names, that child is marked to be what they are called."

And Mama added, "My poor sister Morena. Her fate of what she became was sealed from childhood."

Mama and Papa have a lot of wisdom and understanding, when it comes to life and the reason for people becoming who they are. I still think Aunt Morena should have gone to jail, after stealing from people that have no hands and her own family.

Aunt Heydee takes me everywhere with her; to dancing halls, the theatre, the circus, museums, and art shows. I always look forward to going out with her; it's so much fun. She is my best buddy and friend.

Getting into the circus is a totally different experience than getting into the opera house. There's a lot more pushing and shoving with people that attend a circus. They are common folks and not as refined. When the main door opens, the line of people who've been waiting outside in the cold for about an hour becomes an anxious and agitated serpent of living flesh that is going to push through without consideration for anyone else, even if it takes a few trampled bodies along the way. The idea is to show your ticket to the doorman as quick as possible and run in to grab a good seat. There are no assigned seats, it's all first-come first-served.

Aunt Heydee taught me how to use the mass of moving people to our advantage. The idea is to get pushed in along with the crowd, like riding on an ocean wave. You don't get off until it reaches the shore, which in this case is passing the doorman collecting the tickets, and getting in without paying. This is very exciting, but I got caught once. It was one of those docile, family type of crowds that was moving too slow, and the doorman stopped me and asked the deadly question, "Where's your ticket, Miss?"

My heart stopped and my face flushed hot. I was surprised that he believed me when I said with a trembling voice, "My aunt has the tickets with her, and she is still on line."

He pointed to the side aggressively and told me to wait next to him. I knew I was going to jail; this was going to be the last circus attendance for me. Then a wave of saviors came in pushing through and I let myself float away with them. Before I knew it, there I was seated inside the circus tent, saving the seat next to me for Aunt Heydee.

Twice I had the misfortune of finding all the seats around the circus ring already taken, and I had to go to the very top floor instead. Aunt Heydee and I always prepare ahead as to where we will meet outside if we become separated inside.

The tickets for the last row upstairs are the least expensive and there's a good reason for that. Everybody has to stand up along the rail, crowded with a bunch of other people because there aren't any seats available up there. This is the worst place to see the circus, because it's so high that I can hardly see the performers way down below, and to make matters even worse I always get squashed against the railing by some guy that finds his way behind me and obviously enjoys putting his leg between my legs or pressing his private part against my back. As soon as that happens, I take a deep breath and make a little prayer for God to give me the courage for what I am about to do. Then I reach for my safety pin and jam it in and rapidly out of whomever's leg is becoming part of my body. They automatically move away, giving me a dirty look, but they don't say anything either. I hate when I have to use the pin. I am always afraid they will grab it out of my hand and stab my back with it.

I found out how old Aunt Heydee is. Mama told me how to figure it out, and it's quite simple. You go by the present year; since it is 1961, she is presently sixty-one years old.

Using the Safety Pin.

She is older than I thought her to be. Aunt Heydee would be upset if she knew that I know her age. Besides, she has gone through a lot of trouble to change her age to twenty years younger. All her identification papers, even her birth certificate, show that she is forty-one years old. Mama explained that Aunt Heydee used a special-ink pen to change the numbers.

Winter of 1962

Dancing is where I dream of Alberto. Soon I will be dancing with him. I am allowed to attend Sunday soirees with Aunt Heydee so that I can learn to dance. Mama wants me to learn ballroom dancing, and since she cannot afford to buy me lessons, this is a good way to learn. Aunt Heydee always gets me in for a minimal fee, as she knows the ticket man. I get to dance with many partners. I have no rhythm when it comes to dancing slow while being squeezed by somebody that wants me to follow his steps. I am a terrible dancer, but they don't seem to care, so I step harder on their feet when they hold me too close and press me between their legs.

There is one young man called Leonardo who is studying to be a lawyer, he is very respectful towards me; he keeps a space between us and doesn't squeeze me against him like the others. I dance with him most of the time. He likes me a lot and he said I should only dance with him because he can teach me better since he has a lot of dancing experience. He has been trying to convince me that I am making a mistake by marrying my cousin.

He keeps asking, "How can you marry him if you've never met him?"

I always say, "I have seen his pictures, and he is my aunt's son, and he loves me so I love him too."

I feel sorry for Leonardo because I like him, but he is wasting his time trying to make me change my mind. I am already promised to Alberto, there's no room for anyone else. Besides, Leonardo is not my type. My type of man has to have knowledge of the world, not be afraid of anything; he must be an adventurer that can take me by his side, protect me and love me. He has to be strong yet sensitive, and most of all make my heart speed up every time I see him. I have not met such person yet. I can only dream about him and hope that Alberto fits my expectations, which I know he will since he is an American and all American men are very cool; like James Dean, Robert Wagner and Marlon Brando.

As soon as I dance with a new partner and he starts making advances or asking personal questions I tell him that I am there only to learn to dance so that when my husband from North America comes to pick me up I won't be so clumsy.

Mama told me to say that because I was unable to think of an answer of my own, and at least it is honest. Of course, some of them don't ask me to dance again after such an introduction and that's fine with me, I don't have to hassle them away like some others that don't know how to take "no" for an answer.

The school for brides, as I call it, is just a place to spend part of the day. I find it to be a bunch of unfriendly snobs, and since the first week of classes I'd rather stay to myself. Mornings are for learning to cook, and after the two-hour lunch break we spend three hours learning how to make clothes; following paper patterns, cutting, and using the sewing machines. The sewing teacher has an aversion to anyone that uses a thread longer than twelve centimeters long to sew anything by hand. She says only lazy women use long thread to sew; it's best to have short thread and keep threading as needed. This sounds like a waste of time to me. When she is not looking, I use long thread. I sit way in the back so she tends to forget about me.

I started doing an embroidered white tablecloth with two shades of blue thread and I like it a lot because it gives me something to do besides reading when I am home. Papa says it's really nice work. He knows how to appreciate hand embroider; his family used to have a lace and embroidery business on the island of Madeira in the Azores, where he was a representative for his father's German company.

After the morning cooking class, I don't stay for lunch with everybody else. Instead, I go into the pastry shop around the corner, and with the money Mama gives me to buy lunch at school, I buy my favorite goodies, yogurt and fresh fruits, and I still have change left to use for the movies, to buy chocolates, and for bus tickets back and forth to the airport. I feel very rich.

So far I have learned to make the delicious and world famous *Crêpe Suzette* a paper-thin crepe, flavored, and flamed with tangerine and Curaçao liqueur. The secret to making a "real" *Crêpe Suzette* is in the Curaçao liqueur, which is made with *eau-de-vie*, (brandy) sugar, and bitter orange peels. I already tried three times eating the school lunch made by our teacher, and it made me nauseous. He uses too much butter and cream, it's really nasty. I think that he is French because it's hard to understand him with his accent and he talks fast and his voice is difficult to hear. Pedro the chef is tall and very fat; his white starched uniform is matched with a tall white chef hat. By the time he is done cooking for the morning, his outfit takes on a different look; the apron gets sacrificed first, and then he starts wiping his hands on his backside. I feel sorry for whoever has to wash and starch his clothes everyday. I know how it feels ironing Papa's shirts with starch, not my favorite work. Pedro also wastes a lot of food when he cooks. He breaks the eggshells with one hand and a large portion of the egg whites are still dripping when he throws them out. Half the potatoes he peels are gone with the skins. He cuts the base of lettuces and throws them out; Mama would have a fit if she saw that, as she loves the base of lettuces. He also uses too much butter between the layers of dough to make croissants; and now that I have seen how much fat is put in between the several layers of dough to make elephant ears, I am not eating them anymore. No wonder they charge so much for lunch at the school, it's most likely to cover wasted expenses.

I was walking back from lunch to the bride school when I heard Leonardo calling me from across the street. He came over to me and we shook hands and he invited me to go to the coffee shop with him to sit down and talk. I got all flustered and didn't know what else to do but to cut the encounter very short. So I waved him goodbye as I ran down the street saying, "Got to go, bye-bye."

I don't like to hurt people's feelings, but I really didn't know what else to do but run away from him. I feel so embarrassed because I realize that I have no social manners like the girls I know at school who have boyfriends and are comfortable talking to the opposite sex. I just don't know what to say, and get flustered and confused. I feel inadequate and sad.

Lately Mama and I have been spending more time together. Now that we know I will soon be gone to North America, Mama has become nicer to me and I am starting to feel like we are almost like pals, even though I know better than to confide anything personal with her. We have been going to the movies more often, and today we even went out to a restaurant for lunch. This was my very first time having lunch with Mama outside the house, like a woman-to-woman type of experience. I feel so important being part of Mama's life. It feels good being with her, even though we have different opinions about everything. I don't disagree with her; I simply nod my head up and down at everything. I am afraid to jeopardize our time together.

I found out that Mama's favorite food to eat out is roasted chicken basted in spicy mustard. I liked the chicken, but the wine made my legs go numb, my head felt weird, and it was hard to breathe because my heart started to beat faster and expand inside my chest. That was a weird feeling! Mama said that I am allergic to wine and therefore I should stay away from it. I can't agree more.

Mama can still embarrass me to no end. I have to grin and bear it for a little while longer. I can't really complain since she pays for my movies and she has been buying me ice cream every time we go to a matinee. This afternoon a young man followed us into the theatre. That doesn't bother me anymore. When men follow me I ignore them and they go away sooner or later. This young guy followed us into the theatre and stood against the wall while the lights were still on, staring in my direction.

Mama said, "Watch him disappear from our sight." She removed her dentures both the top and bottom and between her two hands she made them open and close as if they were chewing on their own, *clap-clap-clap*, in his direction.

He opened his eyes shocked and, like Mama had said, was gone and out of sight before we could even blink an eye. Mama laughed and laughed as I tried to disappear into my seat. I felt like Alice in Wonderland looking for a hole in my chair. It's bad enough when she takes her dentures out while having dinner at home and puts them neatly on a white napkin next to her plate.

She says her gums hurt when she chews with them. I think it's disgusting to put your dentures on top of the table where everybody can see them. And she wonders why I don't like to sit next to her. I don't understand how Papa can feel attracted to Mama Linda.

I am getting so pampered. Uncle Augusto's wife Coty invited me to go out with her to the best restaurant in Lisbon to have the latest new drink from North America; it's called "ice-cream-soda." She has never taken me out before. The most experience I have had with her was doing errands from Mama to Aunt Coty's house and then Aunt Coty would give me some fig cookies to take with me so I could eat them on the way home. For a long time I felt guilty because I never told her that I don't like fig cookies. Aunt Coty would ask me, "Did you like the cookies I gave you last time?"

"Yes, they were great," I would say to her, afraid of hurting her feelings; after all, she had told me that they were expensive cookies. On the way home, I would eat the cookie and throw away the fig filling. I love figs but only when they are fresh and juicy, not made into a sugary paste.

Aunt Coty is always home. Sometimes I would find her in the kitchen in the middle of force-feeding one of her children, while they were crying and refusing to eat anymore food. Other times she would be lying down on her bed reading fashion magazines. We never talked much, and in many ways I have always been a little shy of her because she is an adult, married to a doctor, and therefore superior in intelligence and status to anybody else I know. Besides all that, she is Spanish, and her accent makes it hard for me to understand what she says. I have a lot of trouble understanding Spanish. Uncle Abraham's wife Simy is also from Spain but she is not as smart as Aunt Coty, she is still having trouble speaking Portuguese. I hardly understand anything she says.

So, Aunt Coty came to pick me up at home in a taxi and took me to the famous Imperial Restaurant right under the Imperial Movie Theatre. It reminded me of Papa's restaurant with a wide staircase going downstairs and the rooms sumptuously decorated and full of business people having their lunch. Aunt Coty asked me what my favorite fruit was and I told her strawberries.

The waiter brought us both a very tall frosty glass with a strawberry ice cream soda. I thought I was going to die, it was the best drink I ever had.

Aunt Coty turned out to be a cool person; she actually talked to me as if I was an equal. She even confided that once her kids are all grown up, she is contemplating with the idea of teaching French in high school. She wants to stay busy and get a feeling that she is useful in society.

After this get-together I look at Aunt Coty in a different way and I am not afraid of her anymore; she is like everybody else, and a very nice human being.

I lost my friend, the shoemaker down the street. He sits by his window, which is below the first floor and therefore parallel to the sidewalk facing the street where he works, diligently surrounded by shoes of all sizes and colors. There he sits at his small wooden bench from morning until evening, fixing the neighbor's shoes. Whenever he saw me going by, if he was not too busy nailing some heels to a pair of shoes, he would smile at me and we would talk about the weather and his dream. Someday he was going to North America with his family, he would tell me, in case I forgot. I thought he would be happy to hear that in May I am leaving for North America so I took a walk to his shop to let him know about it. But instead he started yelling at me. He had been waiting more than twenty years to get a visa for himself, his wife and three children, to go to Newark, New Jersey in North America, and here I was, a young girl, leaving the country in a few months. He closed the window, cursing me, and I was left there, startled and blinded by tears.

He had never been my friend. All those years I had been a passerby, breaking his monotony with small talk. I am not telling anybody about this. I feel guilty for having told him about my happiness without regard for his feelings. I am ashamed for being selfish. I wish I were already out of here.

Mama took me to Chiado, in downtown Lisbon, to buy an underskirt. The smell of plastic is all over the stores in Chiado, it goes up my nostrils and makes me cough and sneeze, but I still like the smell. Plastic is the new word in the latest household items, like cups and dinnerware. No more cloth hand-embroidered tablecloths either, they are now made of plastic but look so real that if you don't touch you won't know the difference, and besides, they are a lot less expensive. It is the modern way of life arriving to our markets, probably from North America, where everything is made not to last, you use it and then throw it away.

Uncle Augusto asked Mama if there was anything special that I need as a new bride.

Mama told him I need an underskirt. She took me with her to look for the best, most expensive one. She told me that Uncle Augusto is paying for it and he can afford a good one, so we might as well get the best since it is part of his wedding present.

We found one, very, very beautiful. I will be able to use it with any wide dress-skirt and if I am lucky and the wind blows, I will be proud to let it show. I saw others that would have done just fine, and I felt guilty that we were taking advantage of Uncle Augusto's offer, but Mama was set on getting the best, and I didn't say anything either.

Uncle Augusto was shocked and angry when he saw the bill. "This is a ridiculous price to pay for an underskirt. I hope Verónica really enjoys it, because that was the amount of money Coty and I were planning to give her. That's it from us."

I couldn't say anything; as always, I get blamed for whatever goes wrong. I had been blamed for being greedy and the truth is that, even though I did like the underskirt, it didn't mean anything to me. This is the stuff that Mama does that gets me upset. Too bad that I have to take this underskirt with me to North America; I have no intentions of wearing it. It will always remind me of Uncle Augusto being angry for being taken advantage of.

Since the motorcycle accident, Mama has been dreaming about the compensation money she will get from the driver that caused the motorcycle accident. His insurance company should have paid a fortune, but the case was settled out of court last week, and all Mama got was enough money to pay the lawyer and the expenses she incurred with extra drugs and medical bills. I had a feeling about it. I was there when the insurance company had their doctors examine Mama.

I heard them say there was nothing wrong with her due to the accident, what she has now is what she was going to have anyway, since she was predestined to have these symptoms. Being in coma and suffering from blood clots in the brain was not good enough; in their professional opinion she was emotionally unstable and the daily pain and fainting was all part of her "nerves."

How could they possibly know that? Are they gypsies or witches that can read the future? Of course the doctors in our family could not testify on her behalf, it would have been inappropriate. The idea that the insurance company actually paid for all the medical receipts she kept was itself a miracle. But I know that Mama was different before the accident, she never used to faint two and three times every day. Mama has become very sensitive to the touch, her legs hurt, her arms hurt, her whole body hurts all the time, and she is very weak and out of balance and if not careful she falls when she walks. She can also tell when it's going to rain, the broken leg talks to her. She will never be the same; she is to live on pain medicine for the rest of her life. I don't understand her at all, but I do feel sorry for her because this accident made Mama Linda a very sick person, and the insurance company doesn't care.

We keep getting very sad letters from Max-Leão. He wants to come home. He misses us. He says he doesn't get enough food and goes hungry, and in the winter he is very cold. He would do anything to come home. He says it's so foggy in London that sometimes he goes around and around the block and he can't find the door to his apartment. That is what I call British fog.

He had to leave the apartment where he was living because his roommate, the son of the family he was renting the room from, was queer and would not leave him alone. One night the boy even dared to go into Max-Leão's bedroom trying to force him into sex. Max Leão had to fight him off with his fists. Thank God that Max-Leão had a little training in boxing before he left to England and was able to defend himself.

Mama and Papa feel very sorry for him, but they agree that he has to stay in England. No matter how bad it is, it can never be as bad as staying in Portugal without an education or a future.

My wedding is now confirmed for May of this year. Alberto is going to let us know in the next letter as to the exact date. We are keeping our fingers crossed that he comes over in the beginning or the middle of May, and not the end of the month, because that's when I menstruate. We are too embarrassed to say anything and are hoping for a miracle.

The neighbor upstairs got pregnant while she was menstruating and the baby was born underdeveloped. According to their maid, the neighbor's husband was too selfish and didn't care if his wife was menstruating or not. I didn't say anything, but I am wondering how the maid knew that they had sex while she had her period; for that matter, how does the whole neighborhood know that for sure. If that is true, what a mess it must have been, and painful as hell, I am sure.

May is the only month available for Alberto to leave work. He will have ten days off, and he realizes that it's going to be a bit of a rush, but to make up for it we will have a real honeymoon when we get back to North America. We will be going for a whole week to the Pocono Mountains in New York. I didn't know there were mountains in New York. I thought it was just a big city.

Mama has been taking me along with her to visit a few rich people from the Jewish community still living in Lisbon. I feel so embarrassed and ashamed with this whole idea of hers. It's like begging from strangers. It makes no sense. They don't even know us, so why would they lend the dowry money to Mama? We have had no luck so far. Mama is about ready to give up; it will be a relief for me. I hate sitting in the living room of people that I'd never met, and smiling at them as Mama tries her best to tell them how much she needs a loan so that I can get married. Why should anyone care?

I wonder if Papa knows about this project. Nobody is going to lend her money. She has saved so far a total equal to one thousand American dollars and that is more than enough I believe. Whatever it is that she saves by May will have to do. Alberto doesn't need money from my parents because he is already rich; he is an American and an engineer. I think that Mama is worried that without a good size dowry the marriage is off and she is stuck with me.

Mama and I spend more and more time together and I do like that even if I don't agree with her way of thinking and a lot of the things she does. This week we spent a few hours in downtown Lisbon going from one very expensive jewelry store to another. Mama acts like she is very rich, asking the salesperson to show us the most extravagant tiara, bracelet, or diamond ring, and then tells the salesman she is shopping around and will return in another week or so. She needs time to make up her mind, she tells the salesperson. It feels weird to me to waste these people's time, but on the other hand I am with Mama.

   She is always in pain and walking is difficult. Since the motorcycle accident she no longer uses her favorite black high-heeled shoes, only flat shoes made of soft cloth, as they are the only ones she can step in without having calf and feet pain. This afternoon she almost fell when she took a step off the sidewalk, good thing that I was holding her arm and I was able to hold her up. She says she doesn't quite feel her feet, they feel numb. It was lucky for her that I was holding her arm. We take taxis everywhere we go. It's too hard for Mama to climb the steps of the trolley. I am very sad to see what has become of my mother.

I saw Audrey Hepburn in the movie *Breakfast at Tiffany's,* so now I have an idea of what to expect in the city of New York. In North America I will see lots of tall buildings, but also Cowboys and Indians, and I will meet Paul Anka and Elvis Presley and lots and lots of movie stars in Hollywood. I will be speaking English, my favorite language. I will be able to listen to American music all day long, not just at a certain time of the day on one radio station like here. I will be able to listen to the music as loud as I want to and dance to it all the time. I hope Alberto likes to dance too.

I found out that in North America the English language is quite different from the English the British use. I have been learning English incorrectly. Luckily for me, Mama found Lucia, a Portuguese woman who spent five years in North America. I must learn to articulate like an American or Alberto won't understand me. I have been studying American with Lucia at her house now for a month. She also teaches a few American kids, but she told me in confidence that American kids are stupid because their education is below our standards.

Lucia asked me to help her teach and she won't charge for my lessons anymore. That has been a lot of fun because these three kids, two girls and a boy, are real Americans with a real American accent, the way I will be speaking soon, when I am living in North America. She put me in charge of the young boy who is nine years old. I teach him to read English, which is a real joke with my accent; and very basic math, which is simple, so I feel comfortable being the assistant teacher.

According to Lucia, everything in North America is done in a retarded way. The American workers have a low aptitude for multi-tasking: for example, in a factory, when they put a book together, one person gets paid to design the cover, another to put it together, another to set up the pages, another to sort it out; in other words, to put a book together takes more than half a dozen people. Here, one person does everything. I think she doesn't like Americans. There's something about teachers and Communism, every teacher I know calls Americans capitalists, stupid people, and greedy people. I don't know anyone that wouldn't give their right arm for the opportunity of going to North America. I believe they talk down about Americans because they are jealous, and they are the ones who are ignorant.

What a boring day it was. I had to spend the day, the whole day, with Aunt Simy. She is the one who married Abraham, my mother's brother. When she first met Abraham, she was a divorced woman who fell in love with him. She sneaked into his bed one night while she was visiting his family in Portugal, and forced him to make her pregnant so he had to marry her. She is from a very rich family in Spain, but she won't help him with finances or go to work to help out. She feels he is the husband, and therefore it's his problem, not hers. He works as a telephone operator because he had no further education than primary school. He is the only one that takes care of paying the bills. She is too selfish and greedy to part with some of her fortune. Mama and Aunt Heydee always talk about Aunt Simy and how she is mean to her husband. The worst mistake one can make is to get married for money only.

The real story I will probably never know. One thing is for sure, they constantly fight like cats and dogs, and various times Uncle Abraham attempted to kill himself, but without any success. One day, he laid down naked on the kitchen's cold tiled floor, in the middle of the winter, hoping to catch pneumonia, that way she would finally suffer watching him die a slow death, but all he caught was a nasty cold. He loves Communism and gets very excited when he talks against Salazar, our president the dictator. Uncle Abraham is consumed by politics, always talking about politics and the government and how wonderful Communism is and how we should have Communism in Portugal like in Russia where everybody has an equal share at everything. Aunt Heydee and Mama agree that the cause for his bleeding ulcers has to be from burning himself from the inside out. I find his conversation topics very annoying too, and he always has a sad, gray look about his face, as if he were dying. When he comes over to our house, which is rare, I already know he is going to argue about some political stuff, so I leave the room. I can't even imagine how his daughters can live with him. Seeing how the parents are mean to each other, it can't be easy on them.

I am blessed because Mama and Papa are very loving towards each other and they only argue when Aunt Heydee says something hateful about Germans.

Aunt Simy is a short hefty woman with eyeglasses as thick as binoculars, making her green eyes look like two little green dots. This has got to be the worst case of myopia I have ever seen. One of the most annoying things she does that drives Mama and Aunt Heydee crazy is when she walks into our house holding her hand open against her chest and, as she leaves, puts her hand spread out behind her back. It's called *los cincos*; a Moroccan superstition that believes as long as you keep one of your hands opened on your body your enemies will drop dead if they are jealous of you.

Mama and Aunt Heydee take the *cincos* as being an insult towards them, and have been adopting the same motion back at Aunt Simy.

I find this behavior quite childish between adults, but I dare not say anything about it.

When visiting Aunt Simy in the winter, I always find her lying down in bed looking like a seal, wrapped in her mink stole coat, trying to stay warm. She called Mama this week and told her that, as part of her wedding gift, she wanted to teach me how to make her secret grape jam recipe, and today was perfect for her because no one would be home including her daughters who were in school. After I swore to her at least ten times, that her jam recipe would not to be divulged to anyone, and sweating over a stove mixing and mixing and mixing grapes and sugar and grapes and sugar, I was finally let out of her house, five hours later.

My friend Encarnação gave me two very special gifts this morning, a little red handkerchief with mischievous English words printed on it, and *The Bride's Book*. Encarnação made me promise not to show Alberto the red handkerchief until we are on our honeymoon, then he and I can have a good laugh together.

I began reading *The Bride's Book* as soon as I got home. I have been reading it slowly and taking my time to understand each page, which is filled with advice by the expert author. I don't want to miss anything important because, as Encarnação said, this book will teach me how to make my marriage successful. If anybody knows how to make a home happy, it is Encarnação. I only have until May to learn the whole book. It says that as a future wife, I must listen to my heart and the little voices inside of me. They will give me a conscience and the common sense to realize if what I am doing is the right thing to do, because the bride is part of a trilogy with wife and mother!

I am scared, but I have nowhere else to go and no one to share my fears with. I am only looking for love and happiness, that's all.

The Bride's Book is very straightforward. I must always be happy by acting happy and smiling to everybody even when I am sad because men only like energetic, healthy, happy women. This book has a lot of good ideas I was not aware of; like, it's important to cover up our inferiority complexes or sad feelings by forgetting about ourselves and concentrating on the person we are with instead. I must learn to listen and speak less.

That's no problem; I think a lot, but hardly have much to say. It gives advice on how to stay healthy with exercise, and eating healthy, like staying away from fat, fried foods, and sweets. I don't exercise but I do walk a lot, and I have no trouble staying away from greasy, oily food since it makes me sick to my stomach. Staying away from something sweet like chocolate, now *that* is going to be a sacrifice.

The writer also gives a two-page list of the basic needs, to fill a hope chest, like: a dozen towels, a dozen set of bed sheets, thirty kitchen towels, four aprons and so on.

Thank God, Alberto wrote back saying not to bother with that kind of stuff, because he has everything already at home since he lives with his mother.

Mama brought in the seamstress with the bad breath, and she is making me two new dresses to take with me to North America.

I was looking through *The Bride's Book* to find out about the first night of marriage and what that's all about, but it doesn't say anything except two and a half pages of philosophical words like, don't take in your luggage, only dreams of happiness. And, most important, you must not use purple or dark colors in your bedroom; they will take away the brightness of love.

The Bride's Book Encarnação gave me has become my "Bible." Important things to remember from it: When my husband gets home I must have his dinner ready. I should be attractively dressed, smile, and keep quiet until he feels like talking. I must stay graceful and not bring up anything that might get him upset concerning silly daily housewife problems; he has enough pressure and stress with his own job. I must keep his clothes clean and his shoes are to be shined everyday. I must remind him to shave daily and have his hair cut when he needs it, and no matter how hard a day I had cleaning and cooking and taking care of the kids, when he gets home I must be in my best dress, perfumed and ready for love.

I'll be taking this book with me to North America so I can refresh my memory by reading it again and again. If I follow the directions in this book I will have a better chance to be happily married to Alberto, the future father of my children.

I dreamed last night that I had a baby boy with dark curly hair, and he just appeared in my arms like magic. He looked like Alberto's picture, but in miniature size.

Mama said it was a good omen and my first-born would be a boy.

What I didn't tell Mama is that I am very scared of having a baby. I don't know how it's going to come out; I mean, I know from where it comes out and that is what scares me the most. I want to be a mother but I am not looking forward to the delivery.

Chapter Eight

The Way Out

1962

Spring of 1962

Mama was seated in her rocking chair in the living room across from Papa, who was seated in his favorite armchair — because it's not only very comfortable but also belonged to his father. Over the years his armchair started to fall apart, but Mama had it re-upholstered about a year ago for his birthday.

I was walking into the living room and when she saw me said, "Verónica, I want you to sit on your father's lap and make nice to him."

"What do you want me to do?" I asked, scared and embarrassed with the situation she was presenting to me. I had never sat on Papa's lap before, so what the heck was she asking me to do?

"Sit on his lap, and make nice to your father," she repeated with an authoritative tone.

My goodness, I thought to myself, *she has gone completely mad.* But being obedient as I am, I sat on Papa's lap, and stared at her because I couldn't even look at him.

"Touch your father's face with your hand, and make nice to him."

I was scared now. "I don't know how." I said, wanting to cry.

"Just make nice to his face. Is that too much to ask for?" she asked, obviously frustrated.

I stretched my right hand flat, keeping my fingers straight and rigid, and pressed it down on his face as if I was cleaning a chalkboard. Twice I swiped my hand flat, stretched-out across his cheek with my thoughts in a fog as to what to make of the situation.

Mama got hysterical. "Oh my God, what's Alberto going to do with her, when she can't even make nice to her own father. What are we going to do, Joachim? She doesn't even know how to caress!" She was frantic with my inability to show any affection.

No kidding, I thought to myself, feeling like I was going to throw up.

Papa pushed me up and away delicately and said to Mama, "Don't worry about her not knowing how to show affection. I am sure that Alberto, who is an American and a man of the world, and experienced in matters of the heart, will be glad to teach his young bride what to do." And he went back to reading the newspaper.

I felt better after he said that and I quickly left the living room.

Papa hit the roof, when he found out that Mama had taken the tablecloth I had embroidered to a neighbor to have its border done on a sewing machine. He screamed and called her stupid for ruining what he felt was a work of art; the tablecloth no longer had any value.

"You don't sew a masterpiece by hand and then use a machine to finish it off! It's just not done." Papa very rarely screams at Mama, but this time he was furious.

I felt bad about it, because she was worried about my eyes, she didn't want me to lose the little eyesight I have left straining over some silly cloth border.

She yelled back at Papa, "Joachim, the tablecloth is going to get stained over the next few meals and then it will be thrown away, most likely. It's worse for our daughter to ruin her eyes over it, since in North America tablecloths are made of plastic."

Mama is so genuinely concerned with my eyes that she made me put my hands on her head and solemnly swear that when she dies I won't shed any tears. She said that tears are salty and they burn the eyes; besides there's no point in crying over spilled milk, once you are dead you are gone and there's nothing that can be done about it. Crying will be a waste of time, and if I go blind my husband will leave me for a woman with eyesight.

After Papa let out all his steam, he stayed seated on his favorite chair holding the tablecloth in his hands as if it were a dead baby, shaking his head in dismay.

I am glad that I don't have to sew the tablecloth border by hand.

I stopped going to bride school. I am done with housewife education. This week was also the last time I saw Lucia, my private English teacher. She is very excited about my marriage and wants to go to the airport with the family and everyone else to see what Alberto looks like.

I spend the days saying goodbye to my surroundings, the familiar long walks through the parks, taking the boat cross the River Tejo, and the bus back and forth to the airport. I also said goodbye to the front desk people at the American Embassy. No more listening to records of American plays, pop music or light opera and reading their books. I am now well educated in the American way of life so that when Alberto talks to me about theatre or music from his country I won't be completely ignorant.

I went to the temple on Saturday and sat upstairs looking down at the rabbi as he sang with other male members. As always, I didn't understand a word they were saying, but it gave me comfort to sit there and listen. I sat quietly staring at the walls, wearing over my head the old brocade veil that Aunt Heydee gave me a month ago. I felt pretty with it on, and I was hoping that someone would come in and notice how holy I looked with my head covered. I felt the veil gave me a look of religious devotion. I stared at the ceiling and then the empty chairs around me where the women usually sit. The house of God was empty, and it made me sad for a little while, then I realized that the temple was all mine with its warm walls surrounding me and protecting me from the outside world. The future was promising, but I had no idea of what.

I was about to leave when a young foreign woman came in and sat next to my seat. She introduced herself as an American journalist.

This was my opportunity to speak English with an American accent, and so I did. When she found out I was getting married to my first cousin from North America, she took an interest in my life as if I was a very odd finding, and started writing in a notepad my answers to her questions. I was happy to talk to her; after all, I felt like my English was very good because she seemed to understand what I was saying.

After I left the temple I got a feeling that I had talked too much. I decided not to tell anyone about my encounter with the American reporter. If Alberto reads her story in the newspaper in North America before he comes to Portugal, he might change his mind about marriage. Nobody wants to marry a blabbermouth.

We have a new maid, her name is Maria Elena, and she is really nice. She has a very bright disposition, which matches her reddish-blonde curly hair, and she is easy to talk to. Maria Elena knows everything about sex because she is forty-two years old.

A few days ago I was helping her to hang the laundry outside to dry, and she started telling me about her experiences with dating and men and what they want from a woman.

I got this gut feeling that somehow Mama was behind all this sex education so I am not stupid on my wedding night. I am thankful for that, but I whish that my mother was the one to talk to me but of course that is just an impossible wish. I already know how to cook, clean, sew, and even save money, but when it comes to sex I only know what I have learned from the girls at school, the movies, and the romance novels I have read. I've never heard the answers directly from the horse's mouth. I felt comfortable asking her delicate questions because she went into detail about her personal life with different men she had been with.

I was curious, so I dared to ask the forbidden question and she told me that penises come in all sizes, depending on the man, just like some women have bigger breasts than others. She went on to explain how penises get hard and longer than their original soft size.

"How painful is it to put it inside the vagina, and does it have to be that way? Can't it be just kisses and hugs?" I asked, horrified with the idea.

And she said, "If you are going to have children, there's no other way; and yes, most likely it's going to hurt the first time. Some women will bleed afterwards, but after the first time it will be less and less painful until it's the opposite effect and it becomes pleasurable, like when we touch ourselves, but it's even more enjoyable because you share the experience with the one you love." She went on about the wedding night, how I must be helpful and move my body, and even if it hurts I have to endure it until it's over. That's my duty as a wife.

I didn't tell her, but I am more scared than before, and I am hoping that Alberto doesn't like sex.

I got a letter from Alberto; it is now confirmed, he bought the airplane tickets and Aunt Nelly and he will be here for the wedding on May 24. He took that week off from work purposely to come to Portugal. My luck, that's when my menstruation is due, it arrives like clockwork on the 24th of each month.

Uncle Augusto told us not to worry; he will give me a shot of medicine that will prevent the menstruation from arriving that month. I am an adult now, and even though I don't like needles it's a good reason to have one. I only hope it works.

I got a big scare today. I didn't tell my plans to anyone, and most of all I would not tell Mama because I already know how she feels about death. Any time someone dies in our family I am not allowed to go to their house, so that I am guarded from people suffering and crying.

During lunchtime I decided to go to the Jewish cemetery and say goodbye to Grandma Rica. Aunt Heydee keeps telling everyone how wonderful it is to go to the cemetery once in awhile and visit her parents. She even takes a blanket and a picnic basket with her and she sits by their stone for a while, keeping them company, eating her lunch, and telling them all the latest news about the family and what's going on around the world and so forth. I have been there with Mama a few times visiting old relatives that I never met, and her parent's gravesites; so I felt that I had nothing to be afraid of.

I put a few stones in my pockets before entering the metal gates, like I had done before when visiting the cemetery with Mama. "Flowers don't last but stones do," she told me.

I think that stones are also cleaner and a lot more respectful than dead flowers all over one's tomb. I went in and visited Grandma Rica's tomb, and after looking around a bit I found

Grandpa Leão's tomb. The letters engraved in the stone were worn out from so many years of being beaten by the weather. I went around the burial ground, being careful not to step over anybody's graves, and said goodbye to any name that sounded familiar. I left a little stone marker where Uncle Augusto and Aunt Coty buried their first child who died soon after being born.

Just when I thought I was completely alone and was ready to leave, alive and safe from ghosts, I heard a voice calling me, "Verónica!"

I thought I was going to die.

"Verónica!" The same tone of voice rang across the deserted cemetery.

I could not tell where it was coming from; I could not see anyone as the sun was in my eyes. And then again, "Verónica, what are you doing here?"

No ghost would make a question like that after my name. Tthey would have said, "Boohoo." I looked up and it was Aunt Simy, the one married to my mother's brother Abraham. She was visiting her mother Aziza's grave.

I felt so bad when Aziza died a few years ago. A robber followed her home and mugged her before she could climb the stairs to her apartment. He hit her over the head to rob her. She

At the Cemetery.

died on the way to the hospital. I really liked Mrs. Aziza. She was a very beautiful old lady and she was always happy, always smiling whenever I visited her. I wish the robber that killed her gets mugged himself over some miserable *escudos* so he can feel what it is like to lose one's life due to someone's greed.

Aunt Simy hugged me and asked me how I keep so slim, and maintain such a small waist.

I didn't know what to say, since I don't do anything at all.

She reminded me one more time, "Now don't ever give anyone the grape jam recipe. That was my wedding gift to you, and should stay that way."

I smiled at her and said full of conviction, "I promise never to divulge the grape jam recipe to anyone."

And I hugged her as a seal of commitment. I thought to myself, *I don't even like jam, why would I spend a whole day over a hot stove making a pot of jam.* So I hugged her once more and said with meaning, "Don't worry. No one will ever learn your secret jam recipe from me."

May is my favorite month of the year, not just because it's my birthday, but also because the sun makes me happy at this time of the year after a long cold and rainy winter. I just turned eighteen years old, and I know that I am an adult because I am getting married in a couple of weeks. Alberto my husband will be here soon to take me to North America with him. When Alberto and Aunt Nelly arrive, we only have three days to make everything fall into place. I will have to sleep on the hallway floor on a small mattress for those three days because my bedroom will be getting prepared for the reception. Aunt Nelly will be sleeping in the other bedroom up front, which will be especially decorated for her with lots of flowers. That is also the room we are using for me to be dressed in my wedding gown. Alberto is staying at a *pensão*, a cheap hotel, down the street from where we live, until the wedding day. It would be considered in bad taste if he were to sleep in the same house as the bride.

Mama and Aunt Heydee have been making all the arrangements. Even the music to be played at the temple during the wedding ceremony has been carefully chosen so that it isn't too romantic or mushy. Aunt Heydee has put in a lot of work at picking up bright and cheery tunes. She is concerned that the wedding ceremony along with the slow depressing music they always play at weddings might be too much of an emotional issue with Papa, who has a bad heart. According to Uncle Augusto and our cousin Salomão who is the head of the cardiology department in one of the hospitals in Lisbon, Papa's heart is worse than Mama's and they all wonder how he is still alive.

This morning we went to the temple to put together some very important details, like where to put the flowers, the guests, and the tent. Papa came along with us, but he refused to listen to happy tunes for the sake of his heart. He was really annoyed about that, and felt that I should choose the ones I like, since it is my wedding and not his. Of course I picked the happy tunes, as I am not going to be the one to go on a guilt trip if Papa drops dead in the middle of my wedding because of some silly music. I would have to live with that for the rest of my life. I went along with whatever Aunt Heydee had already chosen. Tunes coming out of a pipe organ, my least favorite musical instrument after the accordion, are not going to sound "hip" no matter what is playing.

I am enjoying watching Mama and Aunt Heydee getting all excited as they make plans for the food being served at our house after the ceremony, the car rental, and who is getting the little bags of rice.

Haim, who is Aunt Ligia's little boy, and Rica Gilda, who is Uncle Augusto's younger daughter, will be holding up the tail end of my wedding gown so it doesn't get caught anywhere as I walk up the isle holding on to Papa's arm. I am not supposed to do or think about anything. Everybody insists that I have to stay fresh and cool for the wedding itself. They have everything under control. My job is to relax and enjoy the fun that's coming ahead.

Our house is ready to receive the wedding festivities. The walls have been whitewashed because paint is too expensive. New bright colored curtains have been hung in the living room, and fresh flowers have filled some of the vases that had not seen a flower since they were bought. The whole place is smiling.

It's hard to sleep when the mattress is too thin and the floor is so hard. I was up at 5:30 in the morning. I am wearing the tight sexy pink-cotton American dress that Alberto sent me. I want to look as American as possible. He will be happy to see that I am wearing the gifts he sent, the dress, the ring, and the gold bracelet.

Encarnação took me aside and told me, "I am going to the airport too, and if you don't like him or for any reason you want to cancel this whole thing, let me know and I'll take you home to live with me." She is my best friend.

We all went to the airport a little early to wait for Alberto and Aunt Nelly. Most of our family will be there except Max-Leão who is living in England; that means my parents, José, all my cousins, aunts, uncles, my two girl friends from high school, Lucia, my American teacher, some neighbors, the maid, and best of all Encarnação. In case I have to run away, I can count on her.

I saw Alberto getting out of the plane; he was tall and handsome just like his pictures. He was smiling and that made me feel relaxed, like after taking one of Mama's calming medicines where you are too numb to have feelings or worries. I decided to enjoy each moment as the beginning of my destiny. There was no turning back; my future could only be bright from this day on forward. Everybody was waving and calling him, and then they pushed me to the front of the line. He was walking towards me holding two pieces of luggage, one in each hand. When he saw me, he dropped them both to his sides and ran towards me. He hugged me and then he picked me up in the air as if I was as light as a feather. Everybody started to clap and everybody around me was happy. It was an amazing feeling to be surrounded by happiness all around. I could not ask for more.

Meeting Alberto at the Airport.

We all went home in taxis and Alberto and I held hands and he hugged me a lot, but we hardly spoke to each other. When we got home we got separated. I was taken to Nelly's room where she showed me the wedding dress she had brought with her.

The wedding gown was made of white lace with brocade patterns intertwined with pearls; it was low cut and had long lace sleeves and a long trail. I had stepped into a fairy tale, there was no doubt in my mind, and Nelly was my fairy godmother.

The seamstress with the bad breath was called in to make the gown fit a little tighter.

Nelly had brought many gifts for the family. Everybody was anxious to see what he or she was getting. Alberto and I hardly saw each other, but every time he saw me, he would grab me and lift me up in the air and hug me. I can't wait to be kissed by him on the lips like the movie stars.

At the end of the day, Mama sent the maid with Alberto to show him where the *pensão* was, down the street from our house. I wanted to go with them but didn't dare to ask.

Alberto and I have spent the day running around from one municipal building to another, trying to finish all the paperwork needed before the wedding. We spent the whole morning being sent from one place to another, across the city from one office to another, until someone took pity on us and sent us to the correct address. Alberto doesn't like his name. He wants me to call him Al.

In the afternoon I had to go see a medical doctor to get the okay that I am healthy and I can go to North America. The doctor made me take all my clothes off and lay down on a couch. He pulled the curtain around us and sat staring at me with his little dark beady eyes for what I felt to be a lifetime. He touched my breasts and said, "You are still a virgin, I can tell. So young and pretty and getting married — a child in a woman's body — hmm."

I could feel my face turning red and I was scared that Alberto would pull the curtain and see me naked, so I nodded yes at everything the doctor asked me and stared away from him. That's the way slaves must have felt when they were checked out before being sold naked in the open market. He gave me a clean bill of health and in broken English he said to Alberto, as he blinked an eye at him, "You are a lucky man."

When we left the office, Alberto was laughing about the doctor and called him an old pervert.

It was a busy day, showing Alberto the city of Lisbon, or I should say Al since that's how he wants me to call him. Tonight we are going to a nightclub in downtown Lisbon. I have never been to a nightclub before. It was dark inside and very romantic. The only light inside the club came from the small candle in the center of each small round table. One could barely see much. I felt like a real woman going on a date, except that in my mind I knew that we were as good as married. I was very happy that the tables were small and we had to sit close to each other. I wasn't wearing my eyeglasses. Mama and Aunt Heydee feel that if I wear my glasses I will look ugly and Al will take the next airplane back to North America. Men don't fall in love with girls with glasses. Al talked a lot and I really tried to understand what he was saying, but it was hard to hear with the loud music in the background. So I said "yes" and nodded to everything he said and smiled politely.

They offered us some drinks, and I was surprised to find out that Al doesn't like alcohol even though he is an American. He only likes milk or soda. The waiter was annoyed when he brought us both two glasses of cherry soda. We didn't stay too long because tomorrow we have quite a bit of running around to do.

We have to see the notary, and all the paperwork has to be finished by the end of the day if we are to be married on the 24th. Having doctors and lawyers in the family has helped a lot at speeding up the paper processing, but there's still a lot of leg work.

Our first kiss was not what I was expecting. He took me home, and downstairs he held my face between his hands. I closed my eyes waiting for his lips to seal mine with the passion of the moment. He kissed my forehead and said, "Good night my love, I will see you tomorrow morning." He saw my face and I guess he assumed that I was worried about him getting back to his motel alone, because he added, "Don't worry about me; I remember how to get to the *pensão*." And he kissed me on the forehead again, as if we were friends and not engaged to be married.

I was very disappointed, because I'd imagined my first kiss would be passionate and intoxicating like they describe the kisses between lovers in the books I have read. He is twelve years older than I am. Maybe I am too young for him. He probably sees me as a child, his little cousin. I am worried that there can never be passion between us; we are family, friends, and buddies.

When I got upstairs, Mama was waiting for me at the door. She asked eagerly, "Did he kiss you?"

I nodded yes.

"Was it wonderful?" she asked again.

"Yes," I answered back as I ran down the hallway yelling back at her, "I am going to wash up and get ready to bed, I am very tired," and I closed the bathroom door behind me.

I stood staring into the three half-faces of myself coming at me from the chipped mirror above the bathroom sink. The colorful oil-painted flowers covering the cracks upon my face failed to make me smile. Nothing was going through my mind.

I got up early this morning and was allowed to go by myself to get Al at his *pensão*; we needed to be at the notary by nine in the morning. I was a little nervous meeting a man in his room, even if it was Al my future husband. I told myself that it was okay since we would be husband and wife in two days. I felt that after last night's goodnight kiss I could trust him completely. He does have a beautiful smile; now I understand why as a child the teachers used to call him "Cookie."

He was ready and waiting for me, and he welcomed me with a big hug. We left the *pensão* holding hands, as if we had known each other for centuries. I was full of joy as we walked down to the Praça do Chile, feeling the sunshine rays resting warm upon our shoulders as if it would stay with us forever promising many more wonderful happy days ahead. As we walked down the street I took a few quick shy looks at him, evaluating my situation. I was finally a woman, a real person, and an adult.

I guided him to the *pastelaria* (bakery) down the street where they always have my favorite pastries, *pastéis de nata*, small round pastries filled with custard. I had to introduce him to the Portuguese desserts. It was going to be our breakfast. He ordered two large plates with two samples of each of the pastries enclosed in the glass showcases. I was shocked because there was no way in

Heaven that I was going to eat more than two or three pastries with my coffee. I thought he ordered all that because he was really hungry.

I found out that Al does not drink coffee or tea either, only soda or milk. I sat with glee on my face, staring at the two dishes full of delicious pastries. I was finishing my first *pastel de nata*, when he announced, "We better get going." As it is written in *The Bride's Book*, your husband's wishes are the law. I wanted to put the cakes in a box to take with us, but he said, "No need for that, I'll get you more later on."

What a waste, I thought to myself. Americans are so rich. But I didn't say anything.

When we were running to catch the trolley, Al tripped, and because his arm was around my waist, I fell forward under him on the cobblestones, flat on my face. I was a sore puppy while we sat waiting for over an hour to see the notary. We were announced like royalty as we walked through a long room with palatial gold encrusted walls and huge antique paintings. At the end of the room sat a small, pale, middle-aged man behind a huge dark mahogany desk, definitely too big for him. Al kept laughing about him and saying, "Who is he, the King of Portugal?"

The notary was very dry and would not even smile, as if we were bothering him from more important matters, but he did say, "Tell your Uncle, Dr. Augusto, that all the papers are now notarized and in order. You can leave for North America with your American husband any time you want."

Al kissed me on the way out, right on the lips, not hard, just softly and very loving and it felt perfect. I kissed him back and I was happy.

To celebrate our success, Aunt Heydee recommended a very expensive French restaurant for dinner; she said it was ideal for two lovers. There was a problem though; after three years of French in high school I still have difficulty with the French language, and Al only speaks English. I also found out that his Spanish is as bad as mine, even though he grew up listening to his mother and Mercedes, his Moroccan grandmother, speaking Spanish at home. Al knows two words in French, "oui" and "non," and of course he likes Brigitte Bardot.

It was up to me to order dinner from the French menu. I ordered three different dishes, or so I thought. I never had the experience of ordering food at a fancy French restaurant, actually not even at a regular restaurant. They brought us two small plates of chicken liver pâté with crackers, served on a silver cup. It was okay. We couldn't wait for the next dish. The second order came, and to our surprise two silver plates of liver pâté with crackers was served, this time decorated with a couple of lemon slices around the plate and two olives on the top. Al asked me, "Don't they serve real food here?"

I kept my fingers crossed for the next serving. The waiter commented in Portuguese to me, "You both must really love liver." And he put in front of us two more plates with a small ball of liver pâté surrounded by two thinly sliced pieces of French bread and some parsley on top as decoration.

I had ordered the same stuff three times in different sizes and presentations. We asked for some butter for the bread and left the liver. Al thought it was funny and didn't get mad. I liked the idea that he didn't get angry even though he was hungry. When we got home, I told the maid what had happened and she gave us cow's knuckle stew, the leftovers from supper that evening. We were both starving.

In the morning I told Aunt Heydee how nice Al had been to me when I goofed up at the restaurant.

She smiled and said, "Let me tell you a story, so you are prepared for the reality of life. Once upon a time there was this girl that went dancing and she met a boy in the dance hall. And because this was her first time dancing she was very clumsy and stepped on his feet. She said to her dancing partner, 'Oh, I am so sorry.' And he said, 'My dear, I didn't even feel it. Matter of a fact your delicate feet felt more like a dove flying over mine.' Soon they got married, and after a few years of marriage, about ten years or so, she asked him to dance with her, since it was their wedding anniversary. The same thing happened, she stepped on his feet by accident, and before she could even apologize, he said, 'Maria, you clumsy woman, why don't you watch it, your feet feel like a ton of bricks.'"

Today was spent walking along the River Tejo, and downtown Chiado, and we were on our way home when we met a young group of rowdy Communist students who overheard Al's American accent as he was talking to me. They thought we were both Americans. We had just crossed over the street from the American Embassy when I heard one of the boys say to the others, "Hey, those two love birds are Americans. Let's give them a beating."

Al didn't know what they'd said and I wasn't even going to try explaining to the "teddy boys" that I was not American or translate to Al what I had just heard; I knew instantly that we had to run for our lives. I turned to Al and with a strong look of conviction in my eyes I yelled at him, "Al, those boys want to hurt us, run with me as fast as you can."

He could tell I was serious and started running with me. We ran down the hill like a train without brakes. The boys were running after us screaming, "Yankees! Dirty capitalists, go home!"

We could have won the world marathon as we ran into the American Embassy and told them what had happened. They said things are a bit difficult at present, because of Communism on the rise and with it a lot of ill feelings towards North America. They took us through the back door like we were criminals, and offered to chauffeur the two of us in one of their cars. Al wanted to know if they were going to do something about those boys, but they said it was better left alone, some of those younger people are fanatics and can go to extremes; they didn't look forward to having the Embassy bombed in retaliation.

We got home just in time for dinner. Mama insists we come home for all our meals. Before we entered the building Al bought me flowers, from a street vendor going by our door. I wanted to tell him that I don't like flowers, but I didn't want him to think that I don't like beautiful things. Cutting flowers should be considered a crime, not only because they will die in a few days but also they are extremely expensive. He bought all the flowers the woman was carrying in the straw basket on top of her head; he told me that he felt sorry for her head and now she could go home.

I explained to him that all street vendors carry their goods like fish, vegetables, and flowers on top of their heads. Once you learn to balance the straw basket on top of the head, it is advantageous to have your hands free. I gave the flowers to Mama from both of us.

While we were having dinner, Al got very upset when Mama rang her little metal bell to call the maid from the kitchen to come and fill Al's glass with water. "The maid is not a slave," he said. "She shouldn't have to come all the way from the kitchen to give me water. The water container is right in front of me, I can serve myself."

Al doesn't understand this is part of our culture, we always serve ourselves with water, but guests receive special treatment. Still, I was happy to hear that he doesn't like people to be treated like slaves.

After dinner we retired to the living room area to talk and have tea and cake for a little while and then we said goodbye since it was late. When Al left, Mama caught me in the hallway saying, "Your father wants to talk to you concerning what you should expect on the first night of your honeymoon. He is going to give you advice." Then she called out loud for Papa to come and talk to me, as he had promised her.

His face was one of, Why *am I doing this, I don't want it!* She squeezed his hands in hers as if giving him moral support and said, "Your father wants to talk to you in private," and she pushed us both into one of the bedrooms.

We entered the room and stayed staring at each other for a few seconds. "Verónica, sit down," he said, pointing to the only chair available.

I sat on the hard wood chair by the bed, looking up at him scared of hearing something horrible that I really didn't want to hear, at least not from my own father.

He took a few breaths and then, looking as much trapped as I was, he said, "My daughter, the secret to a happy marriage is the way you sew the buttons on your husband's coat." And he went on, very sure of himself, "Yes, your mother drives me crazy, she can't sew a button properly. Do you know how many times I am at a meeting and the darn button falls off because it wasn't sewn correctly? It is very embarrassing, because it means that my wife doesn't love me enough to pay attention to my needs for the way I look. Use double string, then reinforce it at the end by going around the base of the button, and then secure it with a few tie-ups. How difficult can it be? Do you think that I am asking too much?"

I could understand his frustration with the buttons but what did that have to do with my wedding night, so I said, "No, Papa, you are not asking for too much."

"Okay," he said relieved, "Now we are going out of the room, if your mother asks you if I told you everything about tomorrow night, just tell her yes." And he winked at me.

When we walked out of the room, Papa took off down the hallway. Mama was standing by the door, waiting for me, "Did your father tell you everything about tomorrow?"

"Yes, he did," I said, keeping my fingers crossed. And I kept walking down the hallway just like Papa had done, and hid myself in the bathroom, as I always do. This is the only room in the house with a lock. No more sleeping on the floor, tomorrow night I will be sleeping in a real bed with my husband Alberto, I mean Al.

"Cousin Esther is downstairs!" screamed José as he ran up the steps of our house to give us the news.

I had not seen Esther for a long time. I had my wedding gown on. I grabbed the long trail end of the gown and with everyone else behind me; we all went to take a look. I saw a huge woman, out of breath, trying to climb the steps to our apartment. Next to me, Mama couldn't help saying, "My goodness she is even bigger than I thought could be possible."

"No," I said in disbelief, "that's not Cousin Esther." But Mama was right.

"That husband of hers kept his promise, she sure looks old and ragged," said Aunt Heydee. "He keeps her in the country where she has no other activities but to cook, clean, and have babies."

I met her halfway down the steps. She was out of breath from walking up the steps to the first foyer and apologized for not making it all the way up to our apartment. She wanted to give me a hug and wish me the best. And away she went, back to her husband who was double-parked and impatiently blowing his horn. I felt I'd probably never see her again. It's so sad that people have to change. Life is a happy merry-go-round except when you are on the roller coaster and it's out of control.

In the kitchen, two maids and Encarnação were busy preparing dainty little sandwiches. Encarnação was in charge of the menu and making the wedding cake too. Mama asked me to go to Encarnação and thank her for all the help she was giving us. I hugged Encarnação and said, "I love you. Thank you."

And she said, "It is my pleasure. Go my little one, go, and God bless you. All the food to be served after the wedding ceremony will be ready when you return, but I will not miss your wedding either. I'll be there, see you later."

We had to be at the temple at 11:30 in the morning and then we were coming back to our house where we would have the wedding cake and all kinds of delicious foods prepared for the wedding guests.

The small bridal bouquet of white lilies was very simple but precious. Uncle Augusto decided to pay for the arrangement at the last moment. I have not seen Al this morning. He will be seeing me for the first time in the wedding gown when I arrive at the temple.

After the wedding pictures were taken inside the house, Mama kept her distance from me. A few times that I looked at her she stared at me with a glazed look in her eyes. I had the impression she wanted to cry but her inner pride would not allow it. This was her triumph day. Her mission had been accomplished. There was no time for emotions of any kind except enjoying the moment.

Papa was wearing a black tuxedo and a bow tie. He pointed to his lapel with the small diamond pin I had given to him for his birthday as he said, "I am proud of you, my daughter and remember that this diamond pin you gave me for my birthday will always be very special to me."

Mama was wearing a silvery bluish lace dress with a matching hat. Nelly's pink brocade dress also had a small hat matching the dress, which she brought with her from North America. She and Mama were dressed very much alike and looked very elegant in their outfits. They must have discussed what they were going to wear for the wedding when they wrote to each other.

I walked down the marble steps of our house feeling like a bride should, happy. I took it for granted when I saw a long black limousine waiting outside, and all the neighbors were trying to catch a glimpse of me, the bride. I felt very special as I got in the long black shiny limousine with Aunt Nelly and Papa. Mama told me she was going with someone else in the car behind us. Probably with José, I guessed.

On the way to the temple, I got lots of kisses from Nelly and a few hand squeezes from Papa. I believe they were as nervous as I was. I entered the temple's courtyard holding Papa's arm. Mama was already there. Her car must have sped up ahead. Inside the courtyard I recognized most of the faces that had been waiting for us. Everything had been very well organized; all we had to do was follow directions.

Papa and I finally entered the temple with my two little cousins Palomita and Haim behind me holding the wedding gown's train. There were lots of flowers everywhere, and the

The Wedding.

candles and lights made the inside of the temple look like Aladdin's palace.

Under a white cloth tent in the center of the temple, Al was waiting for me. He had a very serious look about him and didn't smile back at me; he simply took my hand and squeezed it. He looked nervous and he was very pale, probably wishing his father could be there to see him getting married, that's what Mama said afterwards. The rabbi spoke in Hebrew and everybody prayed along out loud. I mumbled, making believe that I knew exactly what I was saying and wondered how many people were doing the same

The wine glass got broken as tradition required. Al and I kissed each other as the rabbi instructed us, and then we walked out slowly to the sound of organ music as man and wife.

In the courtyard everybody screamed in unison, "Hurray for the bride and groom!"

Lots of rice came down upon us. Encarnação was there too, holding a little basket with rose petals, and she threw the petals at us like a prophecy of good wishes coming our way. It felt good to be surrounded by smiles, good wishes, kisses and hugs from everyone. Papa hugged me and Mama did too and then as she stepped back she grabbed Aunt Nelly and pushed her towards me. Then she walked away, just like that. I wanted to ask her to stay close to me but she was gone, out of my sight. She must be glad to see me go; it's okay, I won't miss her either.

Al and I were guided back into the limousine; this time it was just the two of us. Someone told us, "Wait for everybody to get into their cars so we can make a wedding procession."

But Al was impatient, and after waiting a few minutes he asked the chauffeur, "What's taking them so long? Let's just leave them behind."

I didn't have the courage to disagree; after all, he is the husband, and what a husband says, that's what it is.

The chauffeur was laughing, and answered him in broken English, "Usually the bride and groom travel with the guests, are you sure that you want to break the tradition?"

Al laughed back at him saying, "Yes I am sure, let's get out of here."

The chauffeur started the engine saying, "If that's what you want, it's fine with me. I guess I'll be going home earlier."

I was looking forward to the procession, but since there was nothing I could say or do I accepted Al's decision.

When we got home there was nobody there except the two maids hired for the occasion that gave us both a big hug. Then we sat down in the living room waiting for everyone to arrive, while Al kept asking me, "What's taking everybody so long?" Mama and Nelly arrived very upset, but for different reasons.

Mama was upset because she wanted the wedding procession, and of course she blamed me. When I told her that Al was in a hurry, she said, "Yeah, Nelly already told me that Al is a very nervous type of guy, but you are the woman and you must tell him what you want."

In *The Bride's Book*, it says very clearly that the wife respects the husband's wishes, and that is what I did. Besides, I was too embarrassed to say anything.

Nelly was upset because José had lost her movie camera. She asked him to hold on to it because she needed to have her hands free to help me with the wedding gown as I entered the limousine. José got out of the taxi and left the camera behind. There was no way to recover it. No one had informed her that José was irresponsible.

The party was set up in the largest room in the house, which used to be my bedroom, facing the street. I couldn't eat anything except for a spoonful of wedding cake. My stomach was twisted inside-out and the sight of food made me nauseous. Not being hungry made me happy; it meant that soon I would be very skinny like the American girls I had seen in movies and magazines.

Al got into a dispute with Cousin Rafael who was adamant about Americans being stubborn capitalist pigs. I had to navigate Al away from Rafael, who I never liked anyway. I was proud of myself for being able to do that without hurting anybody's feelings. Encarnação wanted to know our honeymoon plans, and I told her Al had already set up reservations from North America for us to get the honeymoon suite for two nights at the most modern and tallest hotel in Estoril. After that we had no other plans. Encarnação encouraged us to take the train north to Coimbra and, no matter what, to go out at night and see the town's once a year special festivity called the Student's Festival. She said it was the best street party anyone could imagine.

Al said that was fine with him. He loves me. He is the perfect husband. I cannot ask for more.

About 3 in the afternoon I changed into my favorite green dress that Al had sent me from America, and we both said goodbye to all our guests. On the way out of the door, Mama handed me a box of pastries and said, "You both will need something to eat while on your honeymoon — it can be very debilitating. I bought them downtown at the most refined bakery. They should last for about three days, enjoy them with Al." And she gave me that *woman*-to-woman understanding look: *Oh my goodness; you may not survive after a whole night of sex and starvation.*

A taxi had been called ahead and was already waiting for us to take us to the train station. We couldn't sit next to each other in the train; it was very crowded at that time of the day. I looked at Al and he had fallen asleep. His head was bobbing around with each bump and sway of the train — *choo-choo-choooo*. I love trains, the way they move like snakes of steel steadily down the tracks. I wondered, *How could Al be sleeping on our honeymoon? Aren't we supposed to be looking into each other's eyes instead? Maybe I am not sexy enough. I know I am not, and will never be like Brigitte Bardot, his favorite actress.* He had a good reason to be exhausted, he had a long trip all the way from North America, and there had been a lot of running around and stress going on. I wondered if he was going to sleep through our honeymoon. I would have to accept that.

When we got to Estoril, Al told me that traveling by train relaxes him, and besides, he was tired. I told him that I understood. And we kissed. I like kissing him.

There it was, the Hotel Estoril, one of the biggest, most modern hotels in Estoril. The bellboy took our luggage with him, but I insisted on carrying my own eight-by-ten-inch matching blue overnight-bag to our room. It was full of essential and personal items; like my eyeglasses to use in case I had to see something from far away and Al was not around to see me wearing them. Some money in case Al and I get separated during the trip, so I could make a phone call or get a taxi. A map of Portugal in case we took the train to Coimbra so I would know when to get out of the train. One extra pair of earrings in case I wanted to change my look. I had everything that was personal to a newly married woman inside this overnight luggage, even a little sewing kit in case something got torn. Tucked away in the very bottom were the unspeakable menstruation towels, four of them, in case Uncle Augusto's shot failed to work. I also had a small perfume bottle, lipstick, and the red handkerchief Encarnação gave me, which I had not shown to Al. I would feel embarrassed if he read the imprinted English words: "Oh, please don't kiss me," the next line is, "Oh, please don't," the next line, "Oh, please," and the last line reads, "Oh," The innuendo is very clear: sex!

As soon as we got inside the room Al said, "I am hungry, how about you?"

I nodded my head and said, "Me too, very hungry."

We went to the hotel's restaurant.

This time I did well; we had a regular Portuguese menu and we both had steak and fries and for dessert our waiter recommended *Crêpe-Suzette*. I told Al that I had learned at the school for brides how to make them, and they are delicious. It's a French dessert and very festive with sparkling flames. The waiter had the dessert chef come to our table and prepare the *Crêpe-Suzette* right in front of us. A real nice show, I couldn't wait to eat one of them. I politely waited to take the first bite until they put Al's crepe in front of him and then we both took a bite. It was delicious!

Al spit the food out of his mouth and into his plate saying, "This is horrible, it tastes like alcohol, have you ever eaten anything more disgusting?"

"No," I said to him, lying through my teeth as I gladly swallowed my mouth full of crepe. Then, to make him happy, I added a facial look of disgust concerning the *Crêpe* dessert.

"Waiter," Al called him over, "We don't like the dessert, please take it away."

"Sir," said the chef, "This is a delicious dessert. How can you not like it, and— what am I going to do with it?"

Al laughed, saying to him, "Take it back into the kitchen and make soup with it."

I thought I was going to die of embarrassment from his comment. I didn't think it was in good taste to offend the proud chef.

Then Al held my hand and kissed it saying, "Let's go to our room."

I got scared with the idea, so I used my feminine charm. "How about a little walk to the beach first?"

I figured, the longer we stayed away from *the room* the better.

On the way to the beach we put our arms around each other's waist, and when I hopped up and down like a bunny he imitated me. Acting silly made him laugh, so I took that as a signal to be myself. He hopped along with me as we walked back to the hotel. I also felt comfortable enough to sing one of my favorite American songs by Doris Day, "Que sera, sera, whatever will be, will be."

Since the first time I heard this song and saw the movie, these carefree words have given me emotional strength to accept my destiny day by day, because life is what it is and that is all there is to it. I was feeling gay, singing, hopping up and down like a bunny, and kissing Al until we entered the hotel lobby and then *the room.*

I went into the bathroom to shower and put on my lacy, white, bridal nightgown and the matching white lacy robe, a present from Nelly. I stayed there, waiting to get the courage to come out, hoping and praying that I would find Al asleep. I was thinking about Nelly on her wedding night. She told us she went into the bathroom of the hotel they were staying in, and when she tried opening the door to come out the door got jammed and her husband had to call the main desk clerk to open it. Poor Nelly, how she must have felt having the hotel crew opening the bathroom door on her wedding night, nothing can be worse than that on your wedding night. I got nervous thinking it could happen to me. I turned the knob and the door opened.

Al said, "I was starting to get worried about you in there, are you okay?"

I nodded "yes" and noticed that he was already in his pajamas.

"We better get into bed. It's late," he said.

I felt relieved when he said that. To me it meant *I am tired, I am going to sleep. See you in the morning.* Still, I wasn't going to take any chances. I figured if I kissed him and said good night before getting into bed it would be reinforced that we were going to sleep. I stood next to my side of the bed and said, "We didn't kiss goodnight yet."

He replied, "Well, get into bed and we will kiss goodnight in bed."

Due to instant panic I became assertive, "No, we should kiss goodnight before we get into bed, that's the way it's done."

He patiently walked over to my side, gave me a kiss and I rapidly said, "Goodnight. I hope you sleep well."

After that, I felt safe and secure that nothing was going to happen after all. He went back to his side and got in bed. I took the robe off and carefully laid it down on the chair next to me — in case I had to get up during the night — and got into bed, covering myself rapidly with the covers.

He started to kiss me and I stiffened up like an ironing board when he tried to remove my gown. I was very scared. He kept saying, "Relax, I am not going to hurt you."

His hands were all over me, and every time he tried to take my gown off I pulled it back on. Then I heard in back of my head Mama saying, "What are you doing Verónica? You are married now. You belong to your husband. You must help him. Don't lay there like a stone turtle."

So I stopped fighting, and when the gown finally came off, he looked at me and said, "You sure have a beautiful body."

I was glad he found my body attractive. I believed he was being truthful.

"We will keep trying each night until it doesn't hurt anymore," he said, "There's no rush."

Still it wasn't a real good night for me. He went to sleep and I stayed awake, looking up at the ceiling. He was a stranger in many aspects, because we had been together only four days, but he was a very kind husband and I felt obliged to stay awake in case he woke up and wanted to try again.

We tried again in the morning, and I was bleeding a little afterwards. Maria Elena had told me it was normal to bleed in the beginning. I wondered if it was that or my menstruation trying to make up its mind to start or not to start.

Al was not interested in having breakfast, and on the way out I grabbed the box of pastries Mama had given us the day before. I couldn't wait to eat them.

We walked to the beach where he rented a paddleboat. We paddled into the ocean and around the seacoast we went. After paddling for a while we stopped to take in the sunshine, blue skies, and beauty of the Portuguese coast.

I started to open the pastry-box. "Let's have a picnic in the ocean," I suggested to Al.

"We shouldn't," said Al, "Most likely they are spoiled from the heat," and he grabbed the box from my hands and threw it into the water before I could stop him. He didn't even look inside the box to see if they were spoiled. I was horrified. All those tasty morsels Mama had gone through the trouble of getting for us had been thrown out like garbage into the ocean. I was sad but didn't say anything.

When we got back to the shore we had lunch at the hotel and then we went shopping. He bought me almond oil for my skin and perfume and the day was a good one. The night was better too, but still it wasn't easy. I love the kisses and the hugs, but I don't like sex. He laughed when he sang, "It only hurts for the first time, and then it doesn't hurt at all…" It must be an American song about losing one's virginity.

We took the train back to Lisbon this morning. Trains sure make Al sleepy. We could only stay for an hour visiting the family since Al agreed to take the next train to Coimbra where we will spend the night. Everybody wanted to know how the honeymoon was going. Al must have said something to Nelly, because Mama came to me and said, "Your husband is having a lot of trouble consummating the marriage because you complain that it hurts. Well, you have to help and get it over with. I understand that it's not pleasant what you are going through, but it is very important that you please him by having intercourse. Now, this is between us, never, under any circumstances, give him oral sex. For once you do that, you will be deprived of intercourse, and it will be your loss."

I couldn't believe my ears. Mama had gone from "ground-zero," sex, to "Let me tell you everything about it, even if you don't want to hear it."

I made believe I was not shocked by what she was saying; after all, I was not about to share these things with anyone, most of all not my own mother. I was afraid she could read my thoughts so I kept quiet, staring and nodding.

I was glad when Al and I finally left, and soon we were on the train to Coimbra. Thank God that I am hardheaded like my father and I don't give up easy. Being half-German gives me an advantage over being half-Portuguese, and decided, *I am not going to allow my husband to think I am a scared little girl in bed anymore. I am going to overcome my shyness and fears and bite the bullet tonight.* Once I make up my mind to do something it's considered done.

It was a long train ride to Coimbra and it was very hot. We were both thirsty. Al asked the conductor going by, "Excuse me, both my wife and I are thirsty, is there any way that we can get two glasses of water?"

"Sure," was the conductor's answer as he walked away. We waited and waited and then suddenly the train stopped at a station. A group of Portuguese soldiers traveling with us got crabby about it. "What the hell is this? Why are we stopping? This train is supposed to be a direct line, what the hell is going on?"

Everybody was wondering why the train was stopping, including myself. Perhaps we were being stopped by a band of robbers out on the track. My mind was racing at 100 kilometers an hour. From outside, someone knocked at our window.

"Open the window!" screamed the man holding a silver tray with two glasses of water.

I was surprised and Al couldn't believe it either. "What a service," he said, "This would never happen in America! Stopping the train just to give us water! Incredible!"

This was my first trip to Coimbra, and I was really looking forward to it; after all, the furthest I had ever been from Lisbon in all my life was to the fishing village of Nazaré. I was curious to see Portugal's oldest University, famous for its romantic students who wear black capes as they roam the city playing their guitars, looking for someone to fall in love with.

After renting a room at a hotel we spent the day visiting the University and its old library, kept as an architectural masterpiece of times gone by. A security guard followed us around to make sure we didn't touch the books. Then we took a walk through the

Portugal dos Pequenitos where the miniature buildings were built like replicas of some of the important buildings in Coimbra. This miniature city was built specifically for children, and unless we are midgets, we can't do much but stand by and admire a city that was not built for adults to use.

Al fell in love with *The Quinta das Lágrimas*, where Inez de Castro was murdered because she was Spanish and consequently not allowed to love the king's son. Al said this was his favorite place. To me it looked like any other country farm, but I told him I felt the same way. What a day. We had a great time!

After dinner I was all excited, looking forward to being part of the street party about to start: the famous Student's Festival. Al lay down in bed while I was getting dressed in the bathroom. Then I heard someone snoring. I couldn't believe it. Al had fallen asleep at the wrong time. I pulled a chair next to the bed and waited for him to wake up; about an hour later it was eleven o'clock. I looked out of the window, and in the distance I could see the fireworks. I finally got the nerve to wake him up, "Come on Al, let's go or we will miss all the fun."

"We'll go later," he said, "Let's take a nap, I am tired."

I lay down next to him. An hour went by.

"C'mon Al," I implored, "We should go now."

He put his arm around me and went back to sleep.

I thought to myself, *here I am in Coimbra and I finally have a chance to see the famous Student's Festival — a once-a-year event, where people come from all over the country to be part of it — and I am in bed. I guess when a man is twenty-nine years old he gets tired easier. I did marry an older man, so I will have to learn to live with it.* I played with the idea of sneaking out; he wouldn't even miss me if I went out for one or two hours. I stood by the window sill for a while, listening to the sounds of the people going by and the festivities in the distance and then resigned, to putting my nightgown on and laying down next to Al, who was still snoring.

I have to accept that I will never be free to do the things I enjoy. I am half-happy for being married and going away from here and half-sad for feeling deprived of being free, more like a prisoner.

We got up early to take the train back to Lisbon. After having lunch with the family we spent the afternoon walking around the city going from shop to shop and doing the tourist stuff. When it started to rain we took refuge inside one of the houses' lobby along the Avenida da Liberdade. While there, we decided to kiss while waiting for the rain to stop. A woman came out of her apartment screaming that I was a whore and should take my man to my own place.

I showed her my left hand with the wedding ring, saying, "Look, we are married, and we are only kissing."

She said, "Yeah, yeah, go home to kiss. My lobby is not a hotel room, if you stay there kissing I will call the police."

Al was laughing and told me he'd never heard of anything so silly. In America you can kiss anywhere in public.

I can't wait to be in America. Al bought a few pottery kitchen items and a huge soup bowl with a cover in the shape of a lobster. Al said it was quite unique and he had never seen anything like it before. I couldn't agree more with him, and I could even add that it was an ugly, grotesque piece of pottery, too big and clumsy; but he liked it, so I didn't say anything contrary.

All the packing is done. Two super-large wood trunks will be going by boat; one for the wedding gown and a few other clothes, and the other mostly wedding gifts, which I am embarrassed to say, were given to us by I have no idea whom. My head has been in the clouds since Al came to Portugal. Everything is moving very fast and the only thing that seems to have balance in my life is being with him. He asked me if I mind that we live with Nelly for a little while until we buy our own home. I thought that was a silly question; of course I don't mind. I think it's wonderful that we will all be living together. I can't wait. I never dreamed that I could be this happy.

Nelly is not going back to America with us. She is staying a few more weeks in Lisbon with the family. Everyone was in agreement that in the beginning of our marriage Al and I should spend some time alone and get to know each other better. Saying goodbye was easy. I was extremely happy to leave Portugal and no longer have to worry about earthquakes. My wish has come true, and I thank God for his kindness.

As the airplane took off, my ears felt like they were going to explode. The pain was so bad that I started to cry. Al held my hands saying, "I know you miss your family already, but I promise we will come back soon to visit them."

I was too ashamed to say that I was crying only because my ears were hurting really bad. When the stewardess came by to ask us if we wanted a drink, I told her my problem. She brought me some chewing gum and that helped a little, until the airplane landed at the island of Azores. I didn't cry, I was screaming. The high pressure didn't bother Al's ears. I was amazed.

While we were waiting in the Açores airport to take the next flight to America, he bought me a gold necklace and earrings made by the island people. When I saw him pay a fortune for it I quivered. I didn't even care for the jewelry, I thought it was too gaudy, but I didn't say anything. Mama told me many times, "When your loved one buys you something, accept it with a smile. Never say anything stupid, like you don't like it; because, after that remark, he will never buy you anything again." So, I didn't say anything except *thank you* and I smiled.

It was a long flight to America, and I believe I fell asleep. I woke up with sharp needle-pain in both my ears, and Al nudged me to look out of the window. I could barely see the Statue of Liberty in the distance; I had to close my eyes as everything was spinning around me. I tried to look out of the window again, and this time we were much closer to the ground, and I saw rows and rows of brick houses with brown ugly roofs covered with TV antennas. I felt as if we were landing on another planet.

I tried to smile to Al, but it was more like an odd, painful-looking grin. I wanted to throw up, and my ears were killing me. I held on to my ears as we landed. I cried without shame. It was the most painful experience in my life besides taking my tonsils out when I was a kid. I will never take another airplane, ever! Al was talking to me, but I couldn't hear anything he was saying, I had lost my hearing. Flying is a horrible experience. Besides, I have no reason to fly because I have no desire to see my family again.

Since Mama made me swear on her head that I have to write to her every week, I will keep my promise, and that is enough sacrifice on my part.

I am standing on America's soil. My wishes have come true. I am looking forward to my life with Al and Nelly, to meeting cousins Ruth and Joe, and seeing the movie stars living in New York City and Hollywood. Even if I don't ever recover my hearing, thank you God for everything.

A READING GROUP GUIDE

Verónica's Diary

The Journey of Innocence

Veronica Esagui, DC

ABOUT THIS GUIDE

The following questions are intended to
enhance your group's reading of

VERÓNICA'S DIARY,
THE JOURNEY OF INNOCENCE.

DISCUSSION QUESTIONS

1. The author refers to her young days growing up in Portugal as "The Journey of Innocence." If you were to write your own diary about your childhood, what would the title be and why?

2. In Chapter Four, Verónica is introduced to religion and is punished for her ignorance. At what age do you think a child should learn about religious differences? Should religion be taught in school and/or at home?

3. Verónica was only five years old when she had her tonsils removed in a most unpleasant manner. Why wasn't she told the truth by her mother?

4. What are some of the contributors to Verónica's problems in being able to socialize with other people?

5. Which events and people in Verónica's era shaped her life the most, and please explain why?

6. How is Verónica unique in her culture and how does this affect her development in both a positive and a negative way?

7. How do the characters in her life story differ from one another?

8. What are the factors that make Verónica withdrawn, and which experiences made her grow the most?

9. In a time period when sex education was taboo both at home and at school how do you think Verónica felt

marrying a man she barely knew? How much do you think the time period in which the story took place controlled the events that transpired throughout her life? What are some of the reasons?

10. What are some of the ways that Verónica's family influences her life, and how do they do it?

11. What were the most inspirational events in Verónica's life?

12. In Chapter Seventeen, Verónica refers to *The Bride's Boo,* as her "Bible" to being a good wife. Considering that it took place in 1962, do you think the advice given in *The Bride's Book* is still relevant today? Why or why not?

13. Do you believe that Aunt Heydee's philosophy, and wild escapades with Verónica, will play a major role in preparing her for marriage?

14. What do you think is the real reason that Verónica wants to leave Portugal? Is it to escape from her parents, to find adventure or to start her own family?

15. How will Verónica's arranged marriage affect the family? Could such a practice be possible in today's society?

16. If you were to ask the author any questions about her Diary what would they be?

If your book club would like to set up an appointment with the author, please contact her at: Handson13@hotmail.com

More about the author - Dr. Veronica Esagui is the internationally known author of the critically acclaimed, *The Scoliosis Self-Help Resource Book,* which includes The Esagui Scoliosis Protocol *TESP* a very specific group of exercises for the spine. By reading this book a person with scoliosis will discover that there are other choices besides drugs or surgery.

Besides being the host of the television talk show *The Authors Forum*, she is also the executive director of The Annual Northwest Book Festival and a member of The Northwest Association of Book Publishers, The Willamette Writers and The National Writers Union. Dr. Veronica Esagui is a successful chiropractor practicing in West Linn, OR, USA.   www.veronicaesagui.com   www.nwbookfestival.com

Jamie Westfall Mansilla - was born in Anchorage, Alaska in 1982. She is currently living in Valparaízo, Chile. She has been deeply influenced by her artistic family and her parent's diverse cultures. Her father is from North America and her mother from Chile. Jamie is also a Yoga instructor and a student at the Bellas Artes Fine Art School in Viña del Mar.
www.flickr.com/photos/jamiewestfall

Danlar - is a professional awarded artist living in Portland, Oregon since 1993. As a self-taught artist since his teens, he has created a unique array of art varying from poetry, photography, sketching and painting. His paintings have been called Abstract Organic; because of the way he captures the earth's innate beauty on canvas.
www.danlarartgallery.com

The Scoliosis Self-Help Resource Book
www.veronicaesagui.com

Coming soon…

Veronica's Diary II - Braving a New World

Much to her surprise, the New World is not what she expected.
But that doesn't mean she doesn't have the tools to survive.

Veronica's Diary III - Awakening the Woman Within

Her children are now grown up; her ex-husband is still her friend,
but her lovers don't fit the role model of the romance novels she
used to read as a young girl.

Veronica's Diary IV - Angels Among Us

Experiencing the darkest days of her life, Veronica is thankful for
the angels along her path, some of who were still exorcising their
ghostly past as they strived to earn their wings.

For information on upcoming events, interview requests and
comments about *Verónica's Diary, The Journey of Innocence,* or
to find out more about other published works, and audio books
availability, please visit the author at *www.veronicaesagui.com*

Request for Pre-Publication Notice

If you would like to receive notice of the publication dates of Veronica's Diary sequels, *Braving a New World, Awakening the Woman Within,* and *Angels Among Us,* please complete and return the form below or contact the author at www.veronicaesagui.com

Your name: _____

Street Address: _____

City: _____ State: _____ Zip: _____

E-mail Address: _____

Website: www.veronicaesagui.com

Postal: Papyrus Press LLC
      21860 Willamette Drive,
      West Linn, OR 97068

Breinigsville, PA USA
06 May 2010
237504BV00001B/3/P